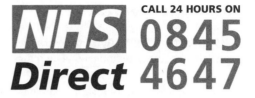

NHS
Direct

CALL 24 HOURS ON
0845
4647

The
NHS Direct
Healthcare
Guide

Dr Ian Banks

Acknowledgements

NHS Direct and **DPP 2000 Ltd** (a joint venture company of the Doctor Patient Partnership, Radcliffe Medical Press Ltd and Software Production Enterprises) co-funded the development of this work.

We are indebted to all those individuals and associations who gave of their valuable time, knowledge and experience to help in putting together this project.

The NHS Direct Healthcare Guide was written by Dr Ian Banks. A practising GP in Northern Ireland, Dr Banks is a prolific writer and broadcaster. The Guide was edited by Jennifer Wells, Sponsorship and Marketing Manager, Doctor Patient Partnership and Jamie Etherington, Editorial Manager, Radcliffe Medical Press Ltd. The Internet version of the Guide was designed by Jeff Conway, Director of New Media, Software Production Enterprises.

To the editorial board who spent many hours debating the format and content of the guide – thank you for your time:

Kathy Agrebi, Nurse Manager, Manchester NHS Direct
Prof Alison Blenkinsopp, Director of Education and Research, Department of Pharmacy Education and Practice, Keele University
Pam Bradbury, Lead Nurse, West Midlands NHS Direct
Dr David Brookfield, Consultant Paediatrician, North Staffordshire General Hospital
Val Buxton, Nursing Officer, Department of Health
Joe Corkhill, Chairman, National Association of Patient Participation
Donna Covey, Director, Association of Community Health Councils England and Wales
Dr Tom Debenham, Medical Director, West Country NHS Direct
Dr Stewart Drage, General Practitioners Committee, British Medical Association
Dr Norman Ellis PhD, Under Secretary, British Medical Association
Dr Simon Fradd, Chairman, Doctor Patient Partnership
Margaret Hewetson, Director of Drug Information, Guy's and St Thomas's Hospital
Dr Rob Hughes, General Practitioner, Greenwich and Bexley Doctors on Call
Dr Terry John, General Practitioners Committee, British Medical Association
Wendy Johnson, Nurse Practitioner in General Practice, Primary Care Advisor to the Royal College of Nursing
Dr Has Joshi, General Practitioner
Bill Kearns, Clinical Advisor to the Medical Director, London Ambulance Service
Julie Knott, Lead Nurse, Nottinghamshire NHS Direct
Kristin McCarthy, Director, Doctor Patient Partnership
Dr Kevin McKenna, Medical Director, North East NHS Direct
Claire Rayner, President, Patients Association
John Stanley, Community Pharmacist, Essex Local Pharmaceutical Committee
Mike Stone, Executive Director, Patients Association

We thank the Consumers Association; Royal College of Physicians; Royal College of General Practitioners; Royal College of Paediatricians and Child Health; British Associations of Accident and Emergency Medicine; and the National Association of GP Cooperatives for their assistance.

Thanks must also go to the following organisations for providing us with the colour illustrations of various conditions: Oxford Department of Medical Illustration, John Radcliffe Hospital, Oxford; Imperial College School of Medicine at St Mary's; The Meningitis Foundation, the National Meningitis Trust; Dermatology Department, Churchill Hospital, Oxford; Dr R Ashton, Dermatology Department, Haslar Hospital, Gosport; and the Science Photo Library. To David Mostyn for providing the wonderful cartoons; John Jago and Blenheim Colour Ltd, Oxford for design and prepress and St Ives Press for printing.

The NHS Direct Healthcare Guide contains general information which can be used as the first step to help you decide the best course of action to take when you or your family are not well. In the absence of any examination, it is not possible to reliably diagnose and treat a medical condition. Diagnosis can only be carried out by a suitably qualified health professional after a consultation. Responsibility for the advice and guidance is solely the responsibility of **NHS Direct**.

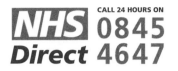

NHS Direct is a new 24-hour telephone helpline. The helpline is led by nurses who can help reassure you and give you telephone advice and health information. Anyone can ring **NHS Direct**, at any time, for health advice.

If you feel that there is something wrong with you or someone you are calling about, a **NHS Direct** nurse will be able to help you and:

■ Tell you whether the symptoms can be managed safely at home and advise you on what to do to treat yourself or the person you are worried about.

■ Advise you if you do need to seek further help from a medical professional and direct you to the right service. The nurse will advise you whether you need to contact your family doctor or go to your local hospital's accident & emergency (casualty) department. In an emergency the nurse can also transfer you directly to the 999 service.

NHS Direct is staffed by experienced nurses who are specially trained to give advice over the phone. They will ask you a series of questions, which will help them decide how serious your problem is.

NHS Direct is part of the NHS and works alongside existing health services. It extends the role of the Health Service providing you with instant access to a qualified nurse who can advise you on the most efficient and effective way to manage your symptoms.

Contacting your doctor's surgery. If you want to contact your doctor's surgery directly either to make an appointment, for a prescription or test, or just for their advice, you should still do so. **Out of normal surgery hours, all GPs operate an emergency service. This service is only for urgent medical problems that cannot wait until normal surgery hours to be treated**. However, if you are still unsure about the best way to deal with your symptoms, **NHS Direct** can advise you on what to do.

The *NHS Direct* Healthcare Guide

The **NHS Direct** **Healthcare Guide** works alongside the telephone service and contains advice on the most common symptoms or problems about which people, day and night, are contacting **NHS Direct** for help. The Guide offers advice on how both adult's and children's symptoms can be dealt with.

In many cases, with the right advice and information, many non-serious symptoms can be treated at home. This Guide helps you decide when it is safe to treat yourself or the person you are worried about and provides tips on what to do. It also helps you to spot the more serious symptoms when you may need medical attention. If there is any doubt in your own mind or if you are still worried contact **NHS Direct** and speak to a nurse for further advice or reassurance.

How to use the guide

This Guide covers the most common symptoms which people call **NHS Direct** for advice. It does not claim to cover all health problems but is a handy reference for the most common symptoms that could effect you or your family. If this Guide does not cover your particular symptom, call **NHS Direct** for advice.

- Use the **Body key** (page 5) to help you find what symptoms you might have. The **Index** (pages 123-28) may also be able to help you.

- Turn to the section of the Guide which covers those symptoms.

- Answer the series of questions that relate to your symptoms and follow the advice given.

- If the Guide directs you somewhere else within the Guide turn to that page and work through the questions in the same way.

- The **Glossary of Conditions** (pages 102-22) will give you general advice about particular conditions.

    The answers you give will prompt you to three courses of action:

     Self Care – it's safe to manage this problem yourself

     Call NHS Direct – the **NHS Direct** nurse will be able to advise you on whether you do need medical attention and if you do how quickly you should seek help

    Dial 999 – you need emergency help now.

Where the Guide suggests looking after the problem yourself, you will be given advice on:

- what to do

- what medicines, if any, you can buy from your pharmacist/chemist which could help

- other people or organisations who may be able to offer further advice.

It is not always that easy to decide whether you have an emergency on your hands or not, which is why you may find calling **NHS Direct** helpful. For more advice on 'What is an Emergency?' see pages 12-13.

NHS Direct on-line

The **NHS Direct Healthcare Guide** is also available on the Internet at www.nhsdirect.nhs.uk You can also find there:
- information about conditions and treatments
- advice on healthy living
- an A-Z guide to NHS services
- advice on health stories in the news.

Use this **Body key** to find your starting point.
What part of the body has the problem?
The colour will then direct you to the section of the
Guide where you will find advice.

Head & chest See pages 14–55

Breathing difficulty in children   *14-15*
Breathing difficulty in adults   *16-17*
Chest pain in adults   *18-19*
Colds & flu   *20*
Coughing children   *22-23*
Coughing adults   *24-25*
Crying baby   *26-27*
Dizziness in adults   *28-29*
Earache in children   *30-31*
Earache in adults   *32-33*
Fever in children   *34-35*
Fever in adults   *36-37*
Hayfever   *21*
Headache in children   *38-39*
Headache in adults   *40-41*

Head injury in children   *42-43*
Poisoning   *44-45*
Sore throat in adults   *46-47*
Toothache   *48-49*
Vomiting in babies   *50-51*
Vomiting in children   *52-53*
Vomiting in adults   *54-55*

Abdomen See pages 56–87

Tummy (abdominal) pain in children   *56-57*
Long-standing abdominal pain in adults   *58-59*
Female abdominal pain in adults   *60-63*
Male abdominal pain in adults   *64-65*
Backache in adults   *66-67*
Chest pain in adults   *68-69*
Diarrhoea in babies and children   *70-71*
Diarrhoea in adults   *72-73*
Female urinary and vaginal problems in adults   *74-75*
Male urinary and penile problems in adults   *76-77*
Poisoning   *78-79*
Adult vaginal bleeding   *80-81*
Vomiting in babies   *82-83*
Vomiting in children   *84-85*
Vomiting in adults   *86-87*

Limbs See pages 88–91

Injuries to hands and feet   *88-89*
Joint pains   *90-91*

Skin See pages 92–101

Burns & scalds   *92-93*
Rashes   *94-95*
Baby rashes   *96-97*
Itchy rashes   *98-99*
Rashes with fever   *100-101*

Body key

How do I know when my baby is ill?

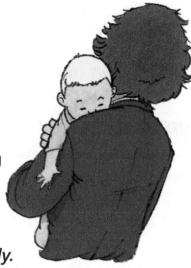

Parents are usually good at noticing when something is wrong with their baby. But it may be difficult to know what is wrong.

Here are some signs that can be important.

1. If your baby is not responding to you normally.

– When awake, your baby may seem unusually drowsy or not interested in looking at you.

– Your baby may not be interested in feeding.

– Perhaps when cuddled, your baby feels floppy or limp.

– Your baby's cry seems different (perhaps moaning, whimpering or shrill), and soothing doesn't help.

If you think you notice these in your baby, please call **NHS Direct** and talk to a nurse.

2. Other signs of illness.

If you are already worried, and then notice other problems too (like those in the list below) – call **NHS Direct** for advice.

– If your baby looks very pale,

– or if your baby seems irritable and dislikes being touched

– or if a new rash starts to appear,

– or if your baby's skin looks bruised or discoloured,

– or if your baby seems hot (feverish, has a temperature),

– or if your baby seems breathless or is breathing much faster than usual,

– or if your baby starts being sick (vomiting).

Remember: you know your baby better than anyone else!
If you are worried, call **NHS Direct** for advice.

When taking a young child to hospital

If you and your child need to go to hospital

– Reassure your child and explain that you're going together to see the doctor at the hospital to make things better.

– Take a favourite toy.

– Dress your child in a coat or dressing gown over night clothes, or take your child fully dressed (it doesn't matter which . . . do what seems most sensible).

– Arrange care for other children or if this is not possible, take them as well (it is unwise to leave a child at home without more grown-up supervision).

– Don't forget to leave a note and take your keys/handbag/wallet with you.

Minor illnesses or accidents can happen at any time so it's worth being prepared. It makes sense to keep some first aid and simple remedies to treat minor ailments and accidents in a safe place in the house.

- Paracetamol/aspirin (children under 12 yrs and asthmatics should not be given aspirin)

- Paracetamol (e.g. Calpol) and/or ibuprofen syrups for children

- Mild laxatives

- Anti-diarrhoeal

- Rehydration mixture

- Indigestion remedy (e.g. antacids)

- Travel sickness tablets

- Sunscreen – SPF15 or higher

- Sunburn treatment (e.g. calamine)

- Tweezers, sharp scissors

- Thermometer (preferably the forehead type for children)

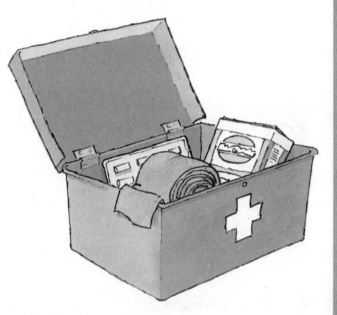

- A selection of plasters, non-absorbent cotton wool, elastic bandages and assorted dressings.

Remember

- Keep the medicine chest in a secure, locked place, out of reach of small children.

- Always read the instructions and use the suggested dose.

- Watch expiry dates – don't keep or use medicines past their sell-by date.

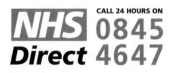

CALL 24 HOURS ON
NHS Direct 0845 4647

We'll take the worry away

Healthy living

Life is to be enjoyed and can be much more pleasant if we were all healthier and lived longer to enjoy it. Simple things can make a big difference and don't mean a complete change in the way you live. Here are some tips on how to stay healthy and live longer, without worrying about it.

Eating for pleasure and health

An increasing number of people are becoming overweight. We know this can increase your risk from heart disease so cutting down on fatty food, especially animal fats, makes sense. Simply grilling food rather than frying will significantly reduce the amount of fat you are eating.

Some foods are known to reduce your risk from many illnesses and possibly even cancer, yet are cheap and taste good. Fruit supplies both vitamins and fibre and can replace sweets for children, especially as a 'treat' or reward. Aim for around five servings of fruit or vegetables each day. (One serving is roughly 1 piece of fruit, 1 dessert bowl of salad, 1 glass of fruit juice or 2 tablespoonfuls of vegetables.)

Try gradually cutting down on salt with your food. You'll be surprised how little you need after getting used to less. It will protect you from high blood pressure.
Fish, especially the oily varieties such as mackerel or sardines, are loaded with special oils which actually protect your heart. Bread, especially wholemeal types, potatoes and pasta are all great forms of carbohydrate which provide energy and should be the main part of the meal. Enjoy your food and go for as wide a variety as possible.

In a puff of smoke

The more we look at smoking and health the more we know that cigarettes are the single greatest killer in our society. Over 300 people die every day from smoking related diseases. Smoking 25 cigarettes a day increases your risk from lung cancer by a staggering 25 times. It also doubles your chances of heart disease.

■ Get someone to give up with you and name the day to start.

■ One day at a time is the best plan, but reward yourself each day by, say, putting the money normally spent on cigarettes in a jar.

■ Tell people in the pub or at work that you are trying to stop. These days they will understand and support you.

■ Get rid of all the tobacco stuff in the house like ashtrays, lighters and matches.

■ See your pharmacist about nicotine replacement which will help ease the cravings.

Go for it. You've only your cough to lose!

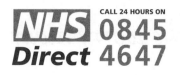

Are you active?

Most people think they are more active than they actually are. Even a small amount of moderate activity will help protect you from heart disease, still the greatest cause of death. Aim for at least 15 minutes every day of activity which leaves you slightly breathless. You don't need to buy expensive machines or even go to gyms or leisure centres.

- Take the stairs instead of the lift.
- Get off the bus one stop early and walk briskly.
- Play with the children. Being a 'horse' for them gets your heart pumping.
- Climb briskly up the house stairs.
- If possible, cycle rather than take the bus or use the car. Most towns are making special tracks for cyclists.

If you are out of doors in the sun, make sure your head is covered and you have a high factor sunscreen (SPF15 or higher).

Sexual health

The UK has the highest rate of teenage pregnancies in Europe. At the same time sexually transmitted disease is on the increase. Using simple protective contraception like male or female condoms would help protect against both unwanted pregnancy and sexually transmitted infections such as HIV (AIDS).

- Condoms are on sale in supermarkets, chemists and obtainable free from your family planning clinic.
- Don't take anyone's word for it, insist on a condom if you are not in a well established relationship. Gay men should use the extra strong variety.
- The emergency contraception (morning after pill) will reduce the chances of pregnancy but it won't protect you from infections. Condoms will.
- Emergency contraception must be taken within three days (72 hours) of unprotected sex. Call **NHS Direct**, your family planning clinic, your local genito urinary clinic or your GP to find out where you get it.

Alcohol

Relatively recently we have found out that moderate drinking for men and women over 40 years can actually help prevent heart disease. The problem is that the message gets confused and there is a temptation to drink too much without realising that this protection is very soon lost as the amount of alcohol consumed rises. To make matters worse, women are more at risk from the harmful effects of alcohol than are men and it's not just a matter of average body size. Aim for no more than 3-4 units of alcohol per day if you are a man and slightly less, 2-3 units, if you are a woman. Alcohol abuse is on the increase and children are drinking heavily at a much earlier age, setting the pattern for later life.

1 unit of alcohol is roughly the same as:

- An English measure (25ml) of spirit. Scotland and Northern Ireland use larger measures.
- Half a pint of normal strength beer.
- One measure of sherry (50ml).
- One small glass of wine (100ml).

Some beers are very strong and we all pour out more generous measures at home. Cans and bottles bought in supermarkets are labelled with the number of units of alcohol they contain.

We'll take the worry away

What are your risks?

Some dangers to health and life are very serious but the risk of actually suffering from them may be very small. These risks can be difficult to work out, especially as the press tends to highlight particular risks to health, making them appear more likely to happen than they do.

It can also be very confusing trying to compare risks. For example, **the risk of being killed by lightning in the UK is 1 in 10 million**. This doesn't mean very much to most of us. So try thinking about it in this way:

At a risk of 1 in 10 million you would need a line of people 10,000 km (6,000 miles) long to contain the single person who would be killed by lightning. It would take 4 months of continuous walking to reach the end.

On the other hand, **the risk of death from smoking 10 cigarettes per day is just over 1 in 100**. The line of people would now only be 100 m (100 yards) long and it would only take you 2 minutes to reach the end.

Reducing risks

Some of the risks to health cannot be easily avoided. Many are so small it makes little point even trying to do so. There are some risks, however, which are not only quite high but also partly or totally avoidable. Cigarette smoking is a good example. Although there is still a risk from inhaling other peoples' smoke (passive smoking), the chances of your health being affected are far, far greater by actually smoking yourself. Another example is the number of deaths from flu which are also small (1 in 10,000) but is higher in elderly and infirm people. These 'at risk' groups can lower their risk by simply having a flu vaccination (the 'flu jab').

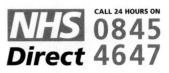

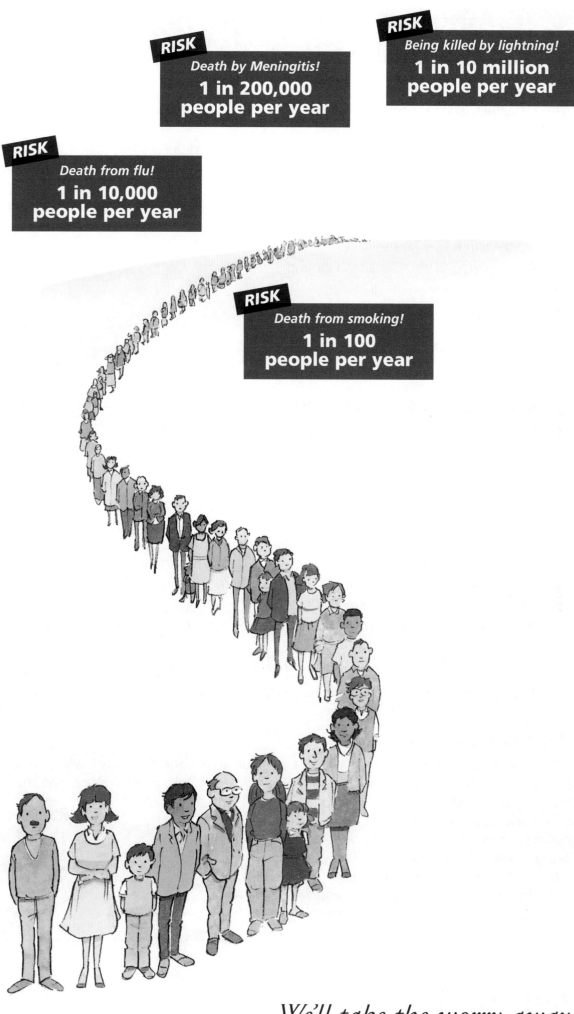

RISK
Death by Meningitis!
1 in 200,000 people per year

RISK
Being killed by lightning!
1 in 10 million people per year

RISK
Death from flu!
1 in 10,000 people per year

RISK
Death from smoking!
1 in 100 people per year

We'll take the worry away

What is an emergency?

When it comes to your health or the health of someone in your family, it is often very obvious if the person is seriously ill and needs immediate emergency care.

An emergency is 'a critical or life-threatening situation'. That's all very well, but it still doesn't really help you decide what a 'critical situation' is. Here are some examples:

- Unconsciousness.
- Heavy blood loss.
- Suspected broken bones.
- Deep wound such as a stab wound.
- Suspected heart attack.
- Difficulty in breathing.

There are a few things that you should remember in any emergency. These will help you to deal with the situation quickly and efficiently:

- Remain calm.
- Do everything you can to help the person, but don't put yourself in danger.
- Don't give the person anything to eat, drink or smoke.
- Don't stick anything in their mouth.

How can you help them?

The way to help a person very often depends on what is wrong with them. Sometimes, the quickest way to help is to take the person to the local hospital's accident and emergency department. This will vary from area to area as it does depend on how close your local hospital is. However, even in an area where your hospital is fairly close, you should call an ambulance and not move the patient if:

- You think they may have hurt their back or neck, or have any other injury that may be made worse by moving them.
- The person is in shock and needs your constant attention.
- The person has severe chest pain or difficulty breathing.

The recovery position

If the patient is unconscious there is a safe position to put them in which allows them to breathe easily and stops them choking on any vomit. Once you have checked that they are breathing normally, lie them on one side, with a cushion at their back, upper knee brought forward, head pointing downward to allow any vomit to escape without being inhaled. Remember when you are moving the patient onto their side, to make sure their neck and back do not move.

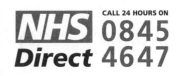

NHS **Direct** CALL 24 HOURS ON 0845 4647

Some myths about Accident & Emergency services:

■ **Accident and Emergency is an alternative to your GP**. *False*

It is not appropriate to go to Accident and Emergency as an alternative to your GP.

■ **Calling 999 for an ambulance gets you to the top of the Accident and Emergency queue**. *False*

Patients are seen based on medical need not who gets to the hospital first.

■ **All injuries need x-rays**. *False*

The doctor or nurse will be able to assess, on examining you, whether an x-ray is appropriate or not. In many cases x-rays are not needed.

■ **Accident and Emergency doctors are more expert at dealing with medical problems than your GP**. *False*

Your GP is an expert in general medicine. A&E doctors are specialists in accidents and emergencies.

■ **Taking pain relief before being seen by a doctor will 'mask' the symptoms of the injury**. *False*

One of the first things that is often done by doctors is to give you a simple pain killer like paracetamol. It is quite safe to take these before seeking advice. Taking pain relief to treat minor injuries is the best way to make you feel better quickly and is an effective treatment. Always follow the instructions on the packet.

Some myths about GP services:

■ **Your doctor has to visit you at home**. *False*

If a home visit is appropriate, the doctor or nurse will arrange it. Doctors decide whether or not to visit a patient at home based on medical need. Only patients who cannot reasonably come into the surgery are visited at home.

■ **You will be seen more quickly if you request a home visit**. *False*

During surgery hours, most doctors visit patients later in the day. It may be quicker for you to go into the surgery both during normal surgery hours and out-of-hours. If you do the travelling, it means that the doctor can see more patients rather than spending time travelling themselves and delaying your consultation.

■ **All infections need antibiotics**. *False*

Antibiotics have no effect on most infections (such as colds, flu and most sore throats) because viruses cause them. Taking too many antibiotics can lead to new bacteria developing which cannot be killed by antibiotics, which is dangerous for individuals and for the whole population. Doctors recommend that you visit your pharmacist for over-the-counter remedies for minor ailments.

We'll take the worry away

Breathing difficulty in children

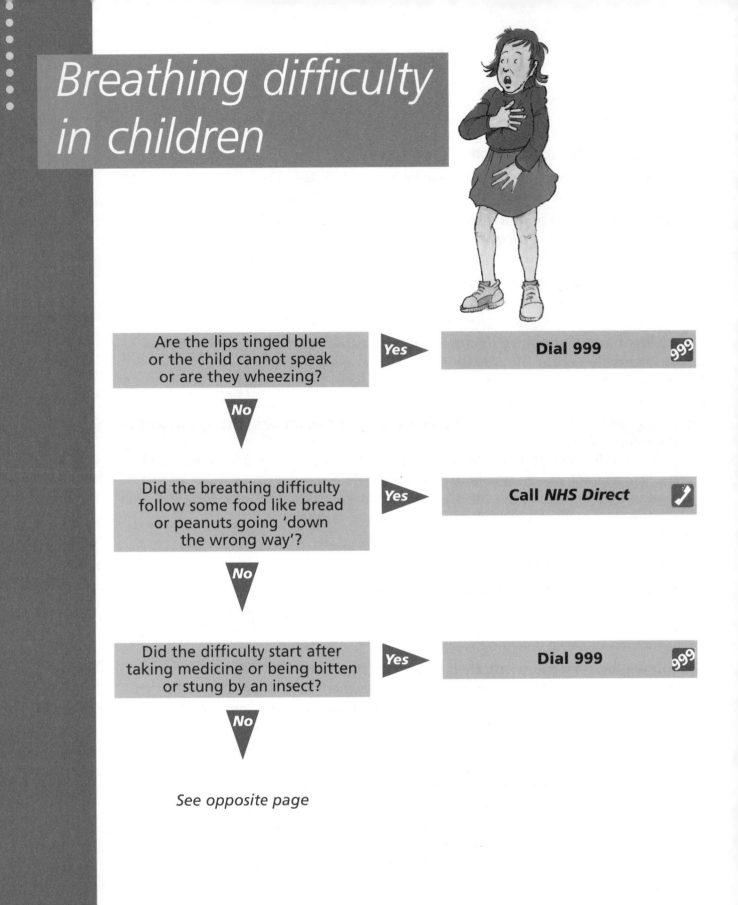

Are the lips tinged blue or the child cannot speak or are they wheezing?

Yes → **Dial 999** 999

No

Did the breathing difficulty follow some food like bread or peanuts going 'down the wrong way'?

Yes → **Call *NHS Direct***

No

Did the difficulty start after taking medicine or being bitten or stung by an insect?

Yes → **Dial 999** 999

No

See opposite page

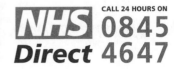

NHS Direct CALL 24 HOURS ON **0845 4647**

Is there also a fever, is the child flushed, feels hot and is sweaty (the child's temperature is over 38°C/100.4°F)?

Yes ▶ | **Call *NHS Direct***

No ▼

Self care advice ➕

- Breathing difficulties in children should not be ignored.
- If your child has asthma, make sure they take their inhalers (bronchodilators) as prescribed and call ***NHS Direct*** who will help to determine the urgency of your child's condition.
- If the condition gets worse or new syptoms develop, call ***NHS Direct***.
- If you are still worried, call ***NHS Direct***.

Breathing difficulty in children

We'll take the worry away

Breathing difficulty in adults

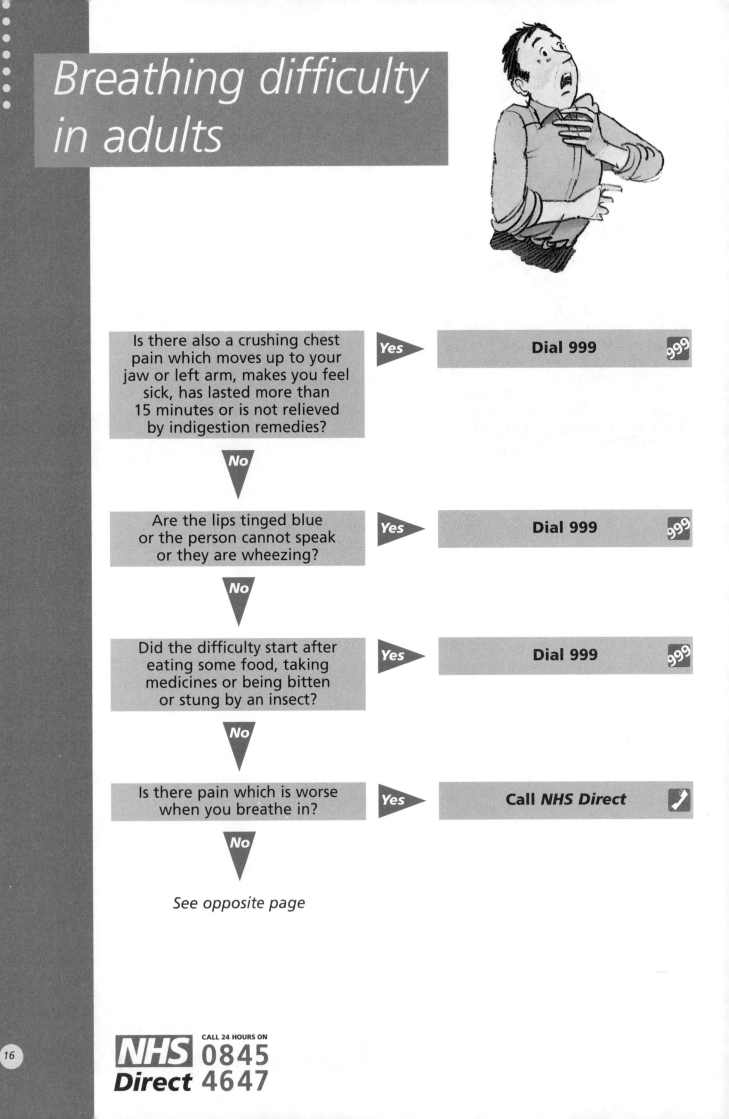

Is there also a crushing chest pain which moves up to your jaw or left arm, makes you feel sick, has lasted more than 15 minutes or is not relieved by indigestion remedies?

Yes → **Dial 999** 999

No ↓

Are the lips tinged blue or the person cannot speak or they are wheezing?

Yes → **Dial 999** 999

No ↓

Did the difficulty start after eating some food, taking medicines or being bitten or stung by an insect?

Yes → **Dial 999** 999

No ↓

Is there pain which is worse when you breathe in?

Yes → **Call *NHS Direct***

No ↓

See opposite page

NHS Direct CALL 24 HOURS ON **0845 4647**

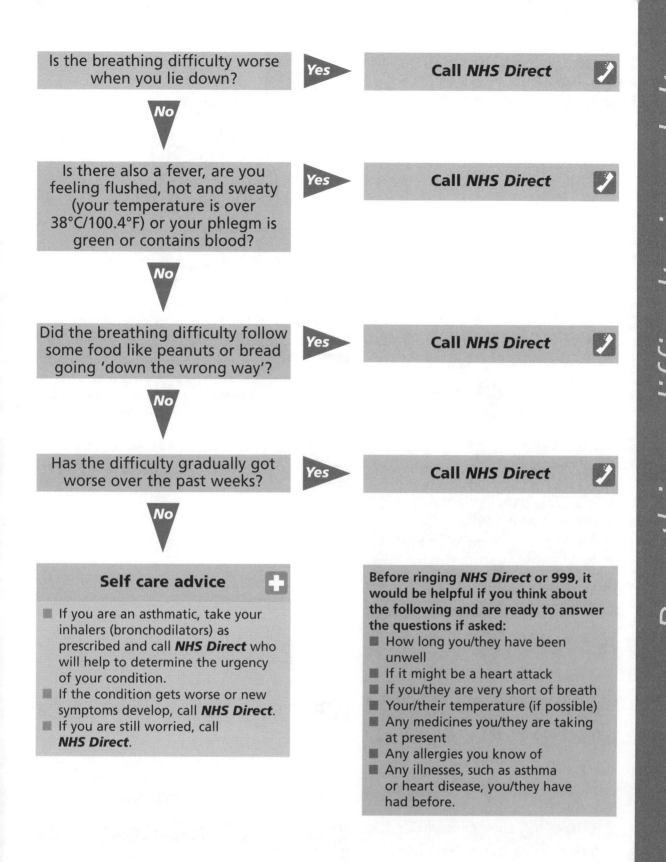

Is the breathing difficulty worse when you lie down?

Yes ▶ **Call *NHS Direct***

No ▼

Is there also a fever, are you feeling flushed, hot and sweaty (your temperature is over 38°C/100.4°F) or your phlegm is green or contains blood?

Yes ▶ **Call *NHS Direct***

No ▼

Did the breathing difficulty follow some food like peanuts or bread going 'down the wrong way'?

Yes ▶ **Call *NHS Direct***

No ▼

Has the difficulty gradually got worse over the past weeks?

Yes ▶ **Call *NHS Direct***

No ▼

Self care advice ✚

- If you are an asthmatic, take your inhalers (bronchodilators) as prescribed and call ***NHS Direct*** who will help to determine the urgency of your condition.
- If the condition gets worse or new symptoms develop, call ***NHS Direct***.
- If you are still worried, call ***NHS Direct***.

Before ringing ***NHS Direct*** or 999, it would be helpful if you think about the following and are ready to answer the questions if asked:
- How long you/they have been unwell
- If it might be a heart attack
- If you/they are very short of breath
- Your/their temperature (if possible)
- Any medicines you/they are taking at present
- Any allergies you know of
- Any illnesses, such as asthma or heart disease, you/they have had before.

We'll take the worry away

Chest pain in adults

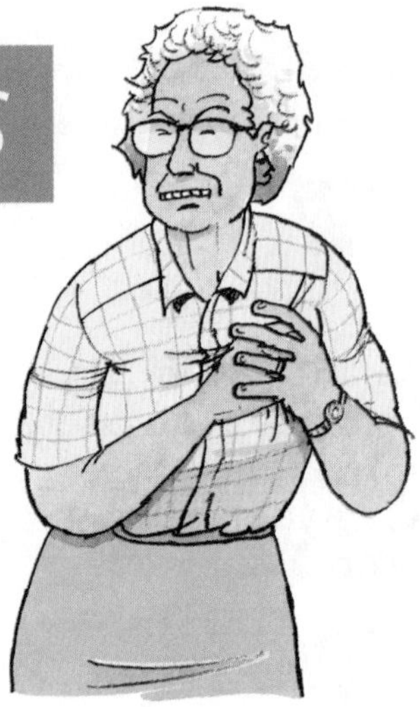

Have you felt this pain before during a heart attack?

Yes → **Dial 999** 999

Dial 999 now. Take any special heart medicines they advise. It may only be angina but let the doctors decide.

No ↓

Do you have **any** of the following symptoms:
- crushing pain like a band around your chest
- pain which moves to your jaw or left arm
- feel sick
- sweating heavily
- short of breath?

Yes → **Dial 999** 999

No ↓

Is the pain worse when breathing in or is there green phlegm or blood in the phlegm?

Yes → **Call *NHS Direct***

No ↓

Is there any shortness of breath or difficulty in breathing?

Yes → **Call *NHS Direct***

No ↓

See opposite page

NHS CALL 24 HOURS ON
Direct 0845 4647

Is the pain relieved by indigestion remedies (antacids)?

Yes ▶

Self care ✚

It may be indigestion. Take any indigestion remedies or ask your pharmacist who will give good advice. If the pain fails to settle within 15 minutes, call *NHS Direct*.

No ▼

Is the pain worse when you bend over and is it eased by indigestion remedies (antacids)?

Yes ▶

Call *NHS Direct* 📝

Go to *Hiatus hernia* page 107 for more information ▶

No ▼

Is the pain worse when you move your arms or have you had unusual or strenuous exercise recently?

Yes ▶

Self care ✚

You probably have muscle strain. **Ask your pharmacist** for advice.

No ▼

If you cannot sort out what to do from this list, please call *NHS Direct*.

NHS CALL 24 HOURS ON
Direct 0845 4647

We'll take the worry away

19

Colds & flu

This advice is suitable for children and adults

Is the person developing a rash that does not fade when you press a tumbler glass or finger against the rash?

Yes → **Dial 999** 999

No ▼

Is there sneezing, runny nose, mild temperature, sore throat, general aches and pains?

Yes →

Self care ✚

It could be a common cold which is not treated effectively with antibiotics. Unless the person is very old, infirm or has some other serious condition you do not need to see your doctor. Take Paracetamol (e.g. Calpol for children), warm soothing drinks and rest. **Ask your pharmacist for advice**.

No ▼

Are you feeling flushed, hot and sweaty? Is there a high temperature (over 38°C/100.4°F), headache, as well as a runny nose and general aches and pains?

Yes →

Self care ✚

It could be flu which is generally worse than the common cold but is not helped with antibiotics. Paracetamol (e.g. Calpol for children), warm drinks, plenty of rest all help. Only groups such as young children, babies and elderly or infirm people who have symptoms which are severe or do not go away need to call **NHS Direct**.
However, if you are breathless or it is painful to bend the neck or if light hurts your eyes, call **NHS Direct**.

No ▼

Self care advice ✚

- Take simple painkillers such as Paracetamol (e.g. Calpol for children) – this will help to bring your/their temperature down.
- Increase fluid intake.
- A simple cough medicine may help a ticklish dry cough.
- Flu vaccination for the at risk group is important. People most at risk: the elderly, people with chronic illnesses such as heart, kidney or lung disease, those with reduced immunity (i.e. HIV or undergoing chemotherapy), and those living in nursing, residential or long-stay homes.
- If the condition gets worse or other symptoms develop, call **NHS Direct**.

NHS Direct
CALL 24 HOURS ON
0845 4647

Hay fever

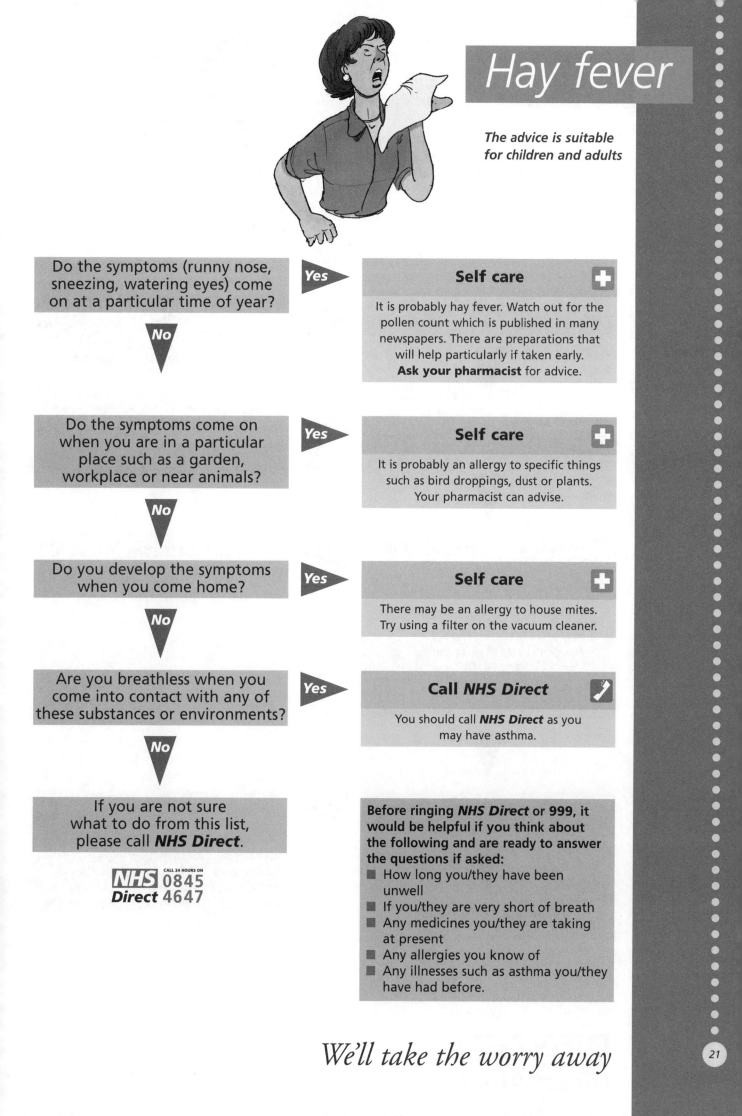

The advice is suitable for children and adults

Do the symptoms (runny nose, sneezing, watering eyes) come on at a particular time of year?

Yes ▶

Self care ✚

It is probably hay fever. Watch out for the pollen count which is published in many newspapers. There are preparations that will help particularly if taken early. **Ask your pharmacist** for advice.

No ▼

Do the symptoms come on when you are in a particular place such as a garden, workplace or near animals?

Yes ▶

Self care ✚

It is probably an allergy to specific things such as bird droppings, dust or plants. Your pharmacist can advise.

No ▼

Do you develop the symptoms when you come home?

Yes ▶

Self care ✚

There may be an allergy to house mites. Try using a filter on the vacuum cleaner.

No ▼

Are you breathless when you come into contact with any of these substances or environments?

Yes ▶

Call *NHS Direct* 📞

You should call **NHS Direct** as you may have asthma.

No ▼

If you are not sure what to do from this list, please call **NHS Direct**.

NHS CALL 24 HOURS ON
Direct 0845 4647

Before ringing *NHS Direct* or 999, it would be helpful if you think about the following and are ready to answer the questions if asked:
- How long you/they have been unwell
- If you/they are very short of breath
- Any medicines you/they are taking at present
- Any allergies you know of
- Any illnesses such as asthma you/they have had before.

We'll take the worry away

Coughing children

*Before going through
the following questions check
'How do I know when my baby is ill?'
on page 6*

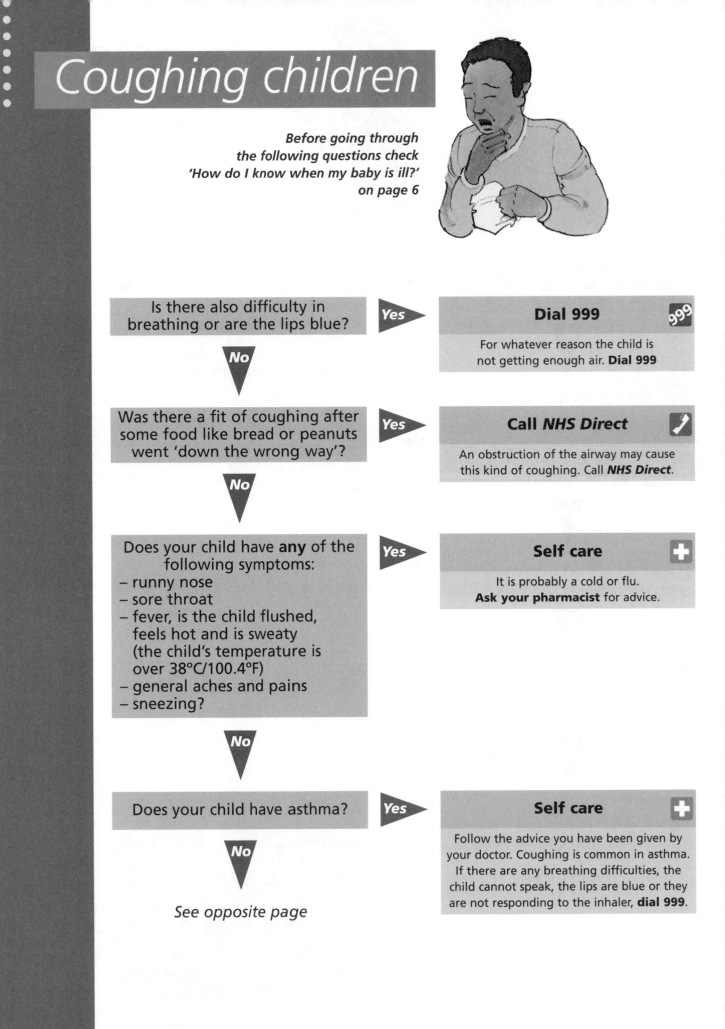

Is there also difficulty in breathing or are the lips blue?

Yes

Dial 999

For whatever reason the child is not getting enough air. **Dial 999**

No

Was there a fit of coughing after some food like bread or peanuts went 'down the wrong way'?

Yes

Call *NHS Direct*

An obstruction of the airway may cause this kind of coughing. Call *NHS Direct*.

No

Does your child have **any** of the following symptoms:
– runny nose
– sore throat
– fever, is the child flushed, feels hot and is sweaty (the child's temperature is over 38°C/100.4°F)
– general aches and pains
– sneezing?

Yes

Self care

It is probably a cold or flu. **Ask your pharmacist** for advice.

No

Does your child have asthma?

Yes

Self care

Follow the advice you have been given by your doctor. Coughing is common in asthma. If there are any breathing difficulties, the child cannot speak, the lips are blue or they are not responding to the inhaler, **dial 999**.

No

See opposite page

NHS Direct

CALL 24 HOURS ON

0845 4647

Is the cough worse when people smoke?

Yes ▶

Self care ✚

Passive smoking affects children even if they are not in the same room as you, especially if they already have some other condition like a cold or asthma. *Either smoke outside or give it up.*

Go to *Smoking & lung cancer* page 120 for more information ▷

No ▼

Does your child vomit after a bout of coughing with a whooping noise?

Yes ▶

Call *NHS Direct* ✐

It could be whooping cough (pertussis). Give Paracetamol (e.g. Calpol) and put a bowl of water in the room to humidify the air. Call *NHS Direct*.

No ▼

Is there any blood in their phlegm?

Yes ▶

Call *NHS Direct* ✐

Repeated coughing can cause small blood vessels to burst. Call *NHS Direct*.

No ▼

Self care advice ✚

- Give the child extra fluids.
- Avoid a smoky atmosphere.
- Home remedy of 1 teaspoon of honey in a small glass of warm water sometimes helps.
- Babies often manage better if they sit up.
- Stay with the child in a warm, humid environment such as a bathroom with the shower on.
- If the condition gets worse or new symptoms develop, call *NHS Direct*.
- If you are still worried, call *NHS Direct*.

Before ringing *NHS Direct* or 999, it would be helpful if you think about the following and are ready to answer the questions if asked:
- How long they have been unwell
- If they are very short of breath
- Their temperature (if possible)
- If there is anyone else in the house with the same problem
- When they last had anything to drink or eat
- Any medicines they are taking at present
- Any allergies you know of
- Any illnesses such as asthma they have had before.

We'll take the worry away

Coughing adults

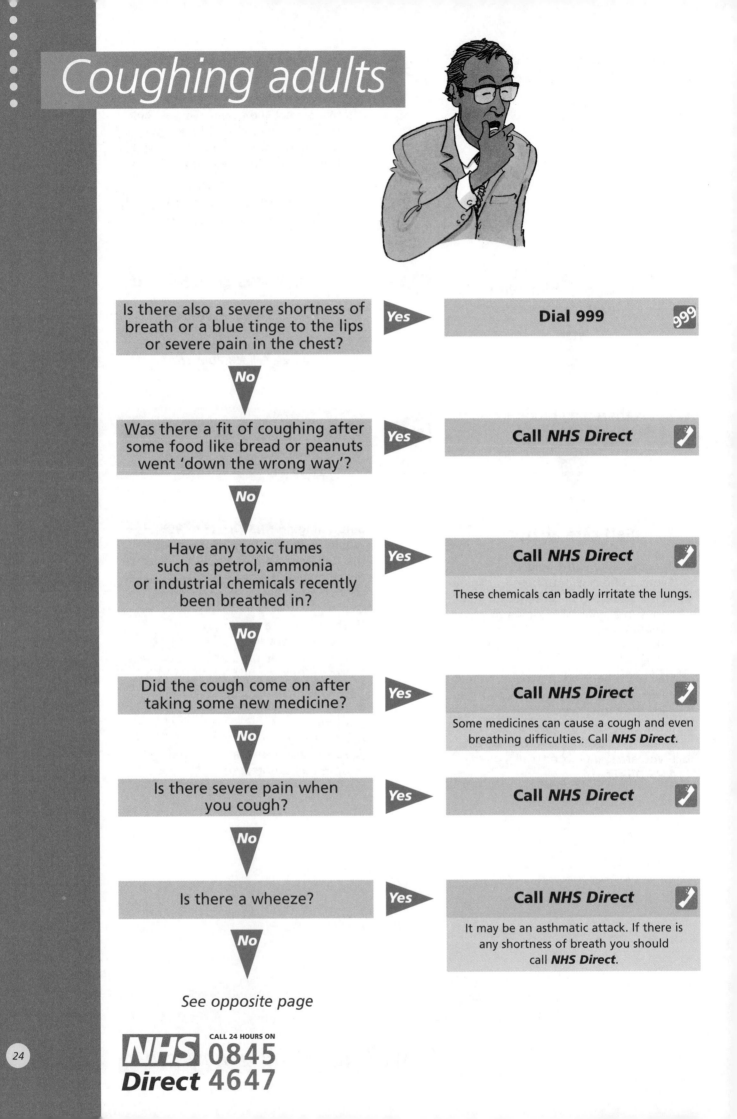

Is there also a severe shortness of breath or a blue tinge to the lips or severe pain in the chest?

Yes → **Dial 999** 999

No

Was there a fit of coughing after some food like bread or peanuts went 'down the wrong way'?

Yes → **Call NHS Direct**

No

Have any toxic fumes such as petrol, ammonia or industrial chemicals recently been breathed in?

Yes → **Call NHS Direct**

These chemicals can badly irritate the lungs.

No

Did the cough come on after taking some new medicine?

Yes → **Call NHS Direct**

Some medicines can cause a cough and even breathing difficulties. Call **NHS Direct**.

No

Is there severe pain when you cough?

Yes → **Call NHS Direct**

No

Is there a wheeze?

Yes → **Call NHS Direct**

It may be an asthmatic attack. If there is any shortness of breath you should call **NHS Direct**.

No

See opposite page

NHS Direct
CALL 24 HOURS ON
0845 4647

Is there any blood in your phlegm?

Yes → **Call *NHS Direct***

No ↓

Is the phlegm green?

Yes → **Self care**

You may have a chest infection. If it persists for more than a few days or you become breathless, you should call **NHS Direct**.

No ↓

Has the cough lasted for many weeks or are you losing weight?

Yes → **Call *NHS Direct***

Some chest infections can last for a long time. Call **NHS Direct**.

No ↓

Is there a fever, are you feeling flushed, hot and sweaty (your temperature is over 38°C/100.4°F), runny nose, sneezing, sore throat or general aches and pains?

Yes → **Self care**

You probably have a cold which will not be helped by antibiotics. Paracetamol will reduce the fever. Use warm honey and lemon drinks to sooth the cough. Cough medicines may be of some value. **Ask your pharmacist** for advice.

Go to **Colds & flu** page 20 for more information

No ↓

Do you or anyone around you smoke?

Yes → **Self care**

Smoking or passive smoking can affect you even if it is not taking place in the same room as you. See *Smoking & lung cancer* page 120.

See *Smoking & lung cancer* page 120 for more information

No ↓

Self care advice

- Take lots of fluids
- Avoid a smoky atmosphere
- Home remedy of 1 teaspoon of honey in a small glass of warm water sometimes helps
- Staying in a warm, humid environment such as a bathroom with the shower on
- If the condition gets worse or new symptoms develop, call **NHS Direct**.
- If you are still worried, call **NHS Direct**.

Before ringing *NHS Direct* or 999, it would be helpful if you think about the following and are ready to answer the questions if asked:
- How long you/they have been unwell
- Your/their temperature (if possible)
- If you/they are very short of breath
- If there is anyone else in the house with the same problem
- If there is bloodied or green phlegm
- When you/they last had anything to drink or eat
- Any medicines you/they are taking at present
- Any allergies you know of
- Any illness such as asthma or bronchitis you/they have had before.

We'll take the worry away

Crying baby

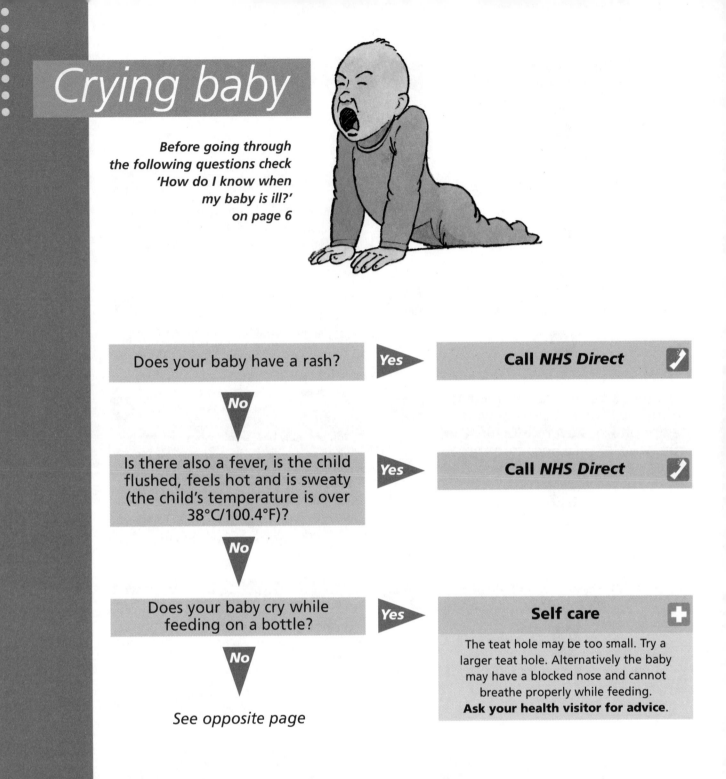

Before going through the following questions check 'How do I know when my baby is ill?' on page 6

Does your baby have a rash? → **Yes** → **Call *NHS Direct***

No ↓

Is there also a fever, is the child flushed, feels hot and is sweaty (the child's temperature is over 38°C/100.4°F)? → **Yes** → **Call *NHS Direct***

No ↓

Does your baby cry while feeding on a bottle? → **Yes** → **Self care**

The teat hole may be too small. Try a larger teat hole. Alternatively the baby may have a blocked nose and cannot breathe properly while feeding. **Ask your health visitor for advice**.

No ↓

See opposite page

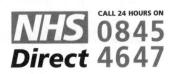

CALL 24 HOURS ON
NHS Direct 0845 4647

Are you able to find a way of soothing your baby?

Yes ▶

No ▼

Self care advice

- If you think the child may be hungry, try to give them some of their normal food.
- You may be able to soothe the child by taking them for a ride in their buggy or for a car journey.
- If the baby's crying does not settle or seems ill, call **NHS Direct**.
- If you are still worried, call **NHS Direct**.

Self care

Your baby may have Colic. No one knows the cause of Colic. It is not due to bad parenting but parents often feel they must be doing something wrong. Gentle soothing and rocking may help your baby relax and settle down. Once the baby has stopped crying and is drowsy, put the baby down to sleep. If your baby starts crying again, leave them for 10–15 minutes before trying soothing again. Although crying can be reduced, it is much easier to cope with if it can be shared. Even if you can't get someone to help you at home try to talk about your feelings. Your doctor, practice nurse or health visitor will understand how hard it can be to deal with a crying baby who is otherwise healthy and well.

Crying baby

We'll take the worry away

Dizziness in adults

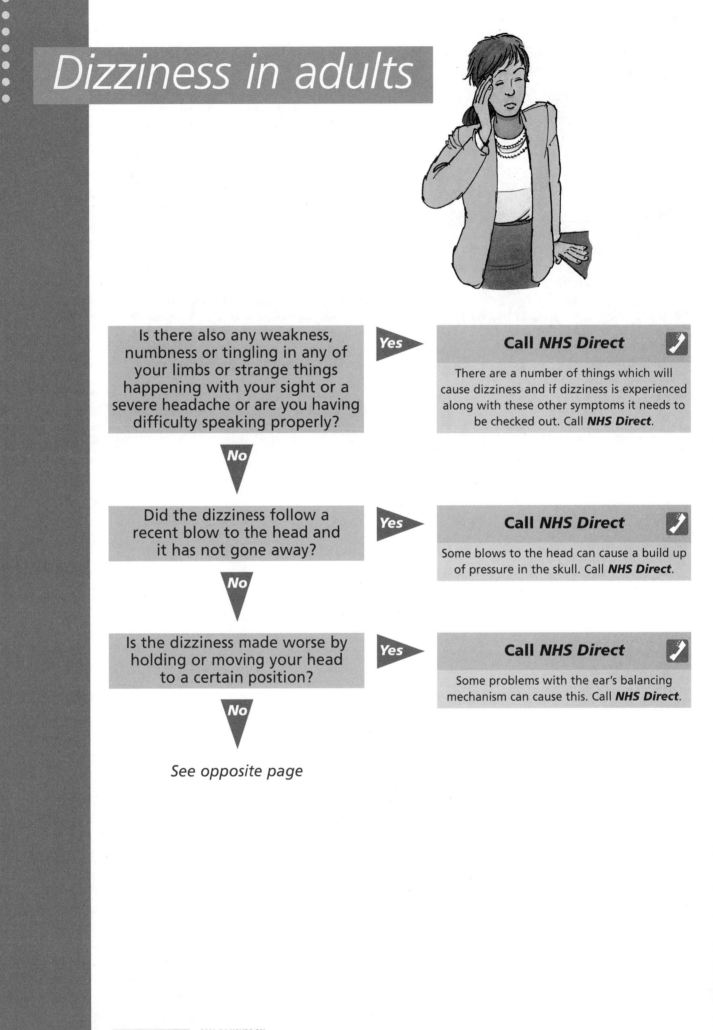

Is there also any weakness, numbness or tingling in any of your limbs or strange things happening with your sight or a severe headache or are you having difficulty speaking properly?

Yes ▶ **Call *NHS Direct***

There are a number of things which will cause dizziness and if dizziness is experienced along with these other symptoms it needs to be checked out. Call ***NHS Direct***.

▼ **No**

Did the dizziness follow a recent blow to the head and it has not gone away?

Yes ▶ **Call *NHS Direct***

Some blows to the head can cause a build up of pressure in the skull. Call ***NHS Direct***.

▼ **No**

Is the dizziness made worse by holding or moving your head to a certain position?

Yes ▶ **Call *NHS Direct***

Some problems with the ear's balancing mechanism can cause this. Call ***NHS Direct***.

▼ **No**

See opposite page

NHS Direct CALL 24 HOURS ON **0845 4647**

Is there pain in the ear or loss of hearing or a strange noise which won't go away?

Yes

Call *NHS Direct*

Some ear infections will cause these effects. Call *NHS Direct*.

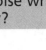 **No**

Self care advice ✚

- Take things very carefully – try not to make sudden movements.
- The person with dizziness should not drive a vehicle.
- If the condition gets worse or new symptoms develop, call *NHS Direct*.
- If you are still worried, call *NHS Direct*.

Before ringing *NHS Direct* or 999, it would be helpful if you think about the following and are ready to answer the questions if asked:

- How long you/they have been unwell and did it follow a recent head injury
- If there is any weakness or change in feeling in any limbs
- Your/their temperature (if possible)
- If there is any neck pain
- If there is any pain in the ear
- If you/they are confused, drowsy or vomiting
- If there is anyone else in the house with the same problem
- When you/they last had anything to drink or eat
- Any medicines you/they are taking at present
- Any illnesses such as ear infections, which you/they have had before.

We'll take the worry away

Earache in children

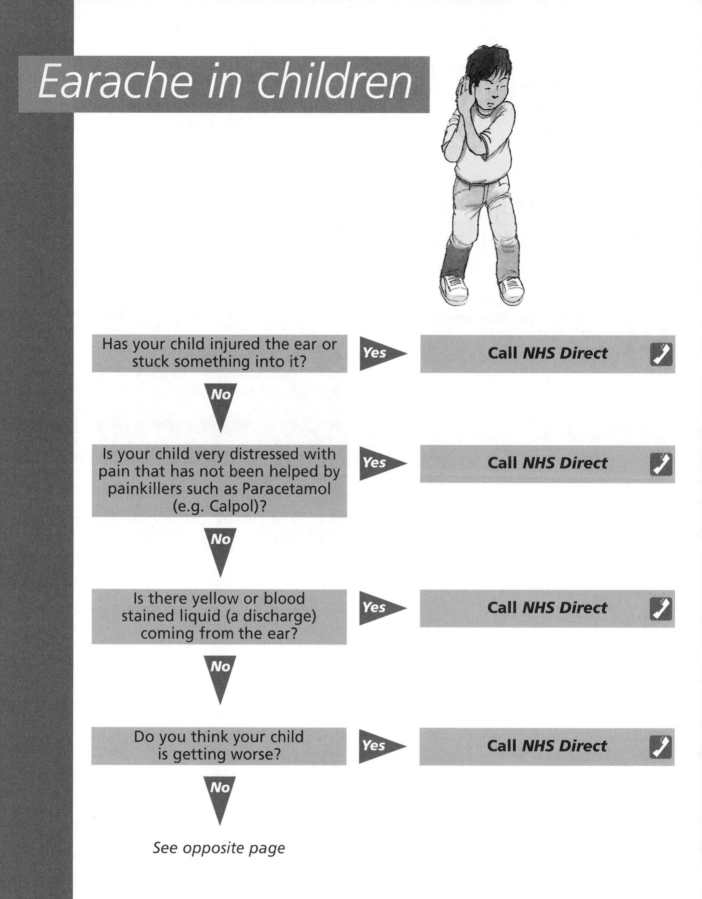

Has your child injured the ear or stuck something into it?

Yes ▶ Call *NHS Direct*

No ▼

Is your child very distressed with pain that has not been helped by painkillers such as Paracetamol (e.g. Calpol)?

Yes ▶ Call *NHS Direct*

No ▼

Is there yellow or blood stained liquid (a discharge) coming from the ear?

Yes ▶ Call *NHS Direct*

No ▼

Do you think your child is getting worse?

Yes ▶ Call *NHS Direct*

No ▼

See opposite page

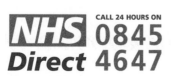

NHS Direct CALL 24 HOURS ON **0845 4647**

Has the child got lumps behind the ear? **Yes** ▶ **Call *NHS Direct***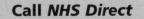

No ▼

Self care advice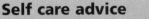

Earache is a common and unpleasant symptom in childhood.

Most ear infections will clear up on their own but there are ways you can help relieve the symptoms:

- A painkiller such as children's Paracetamol (e.g. Calpol, maximum suggested dosage) will help relieve the pain.
- Place your child in an upright position with pillows.
- A warm hot water bottle wrapped in a towel placed over the infected ear may give some pain relief.
- Keep your child away from smoky environments.
- Don't let your child drink from a bottle while lying down.
- Don't bother to give decongestants they will not help to relieve symptoms.
- Never poke any objects into the ear (e.g. cotton buds), they often tend to impact wax and can damage the ear.
- If the condition gets worse or new symptoms develop, call ***NHS Direct***.
- If you are still worried, call ***NHS Direct***.

We'll take the worry away

Earache in adults

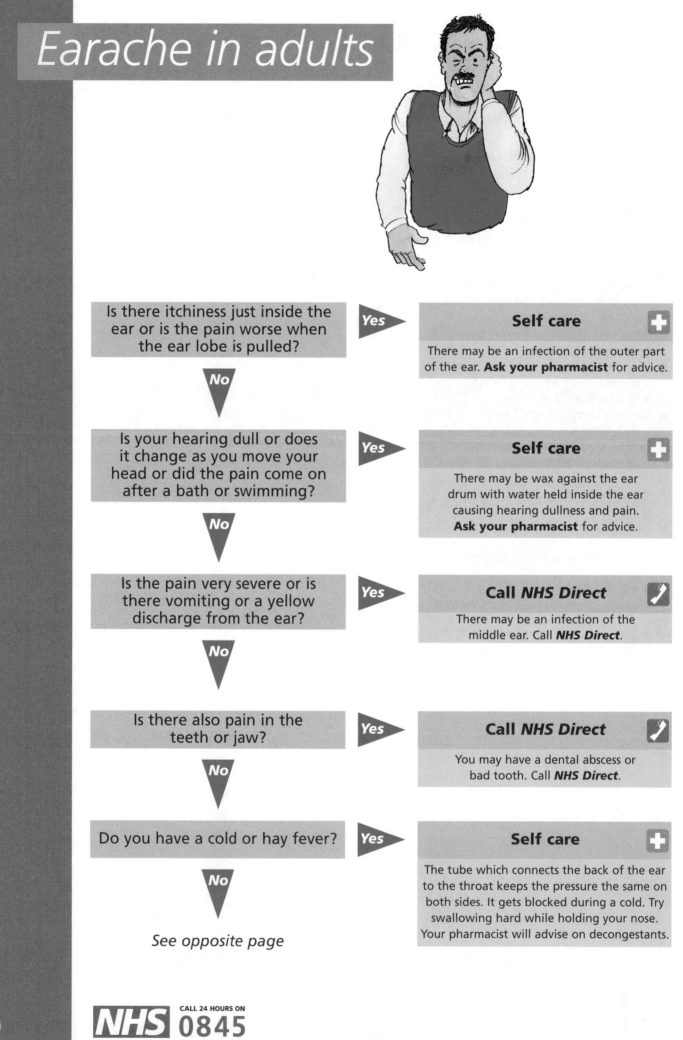

Is there itchiness just inside the ear or is the pain worse when the ear lobe is pulled?

Yes →

Self care ✚

There may be an infection of the outer part of the ear. **Ask your pharmacist** for advice.

No ↓

Is your hearing dull or does it change as you move your head or did the pain come on after a bath or swimming?

Yes →

Self care ✚

There may be wax against the ear drum with water held inside the ear causing hearing dullness and pain. **Ask your pharmacist** for advice.

No ↓

Is the pain very severe or is there vomiting or a yellow discharge from the ear?

Yes →

Call *NHS Direct*

There may be an infection of the middle ear. Call **NHS Direct**.

No ↓

Is there also pain in the teeth or jaw?

Yes →

Call *NHS Direct*

You may have a dental abscess or bad tooth. Call **NHS Direct**.

No ↓

Do you have a cold or hay fever?

Yes →

Self care ✚

The tube which connects the back of the ear to the throat keeps the pressure the same on both sides. It gets blocked during a cold. Try swallowing hard while holding your nose. Your pharmacist will advise on decongestants.

No ↓

See opposite page

NHS Direct

CALL 24 HOURS ON
0845 4647

Did the pain come on during or after a plane trip?

Yes ►

Self care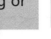

There may have been unequal pressure on each side of the eardrum. This happens more often when you have a cold or an ear infection. Try swallowing hard while holding your nose. Take Paracetamol. **If the pain does not go away after two days speak to your doctor.**

No ▼

Did the pain come on after trying to clean out wax with your finger or some object?

Yes ►

Call *NHS Direct*

You may have damaged the sensitive lining of the ear or even the eardrum itself. The smallest thing you should put in your ear is your elbow! Never use cotton buds to clear wax as they only push the wax further in and may cause damage to the inside of your ear.

No ▼

Self care advice

- Try simple painkillers.
- If the cold/wind makes your earache worse, cover yor ears with hat/scarf.
- If the condition gets worse or new symptoms develop, call **NHS Direct**.
- If you are still worried, call **NHS Direct**.

We'll take the worry away

Fever in children

Your child may have a fever, if he/she is flushed, feels hot and is sweaty (their temperature is over 38°C/100.4°F)

Is your child under 1 year old? **Yes** → **Call NHS Direct**

No ↓

Is there a rash? **Yes** → Go to *Rashes with fever* page 100 for more information

No ↓

Are there any tender swellings around the jaw and neck? **Yes** → **Self care**

It is probably swollen glands. Give the child Paracetamol (e.g. Calpol) and plenty of cool drinks and **ask your pharmacist** for advice. If the symptoms continue speak to your doctor.

No ↓

Is there earache? **Yes** → Go to *Earache in children* page 30 for more information

No ↓

Is there a sore throat or sneezing or a cough or a runny nose? **Yes** → **Self care**

It is probably a cold or flu. **Ask your pharmacist** for advice.

No ↓

Is there also diarrhoea? **Yes** → Go to *Diarrhoea in babies and children* page 70 for more information

No ↓

See opposite page

NHS Direct CALL 24 HOURS ON **0845 4647**

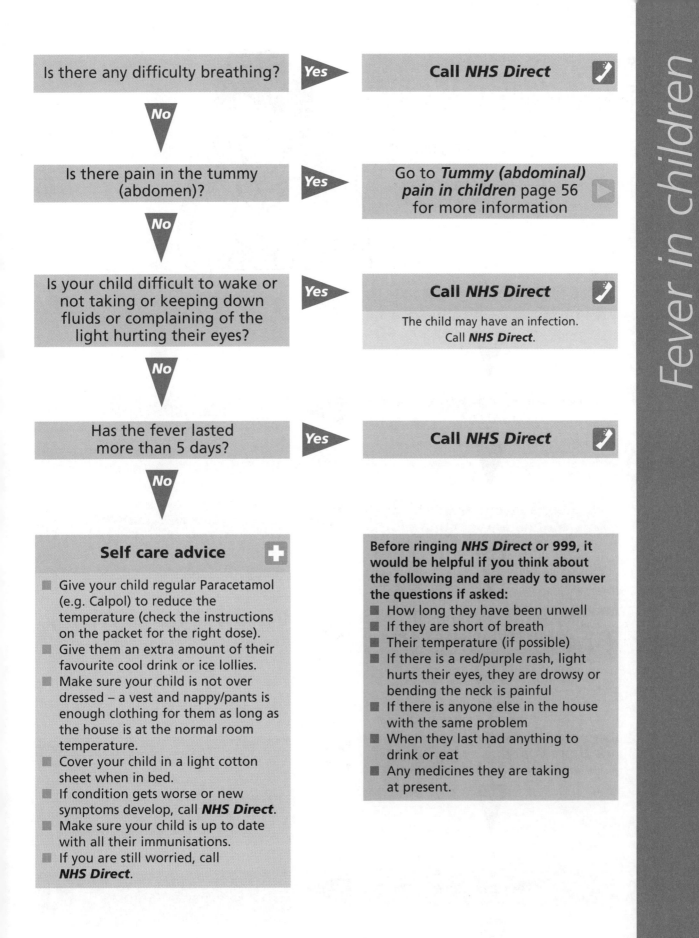

Is there any difficulty breathing? **Yes** → **Call _NHS Direct_**

No ↓

Is there pain in the tummy (abdomen)? **Yes** → Go to _Tummy (abdominal) pain in children_ page 56 for more information

No ↓

Is your child difficult to wake or not taking or keeping down fluids or complaining of the light hurting their eyes? **Yes** → **Call _NHS Direct_**

The child may have an infection. Call _NHS Direct_.

No ↓

Has the fever lasted more than 5 days? **Yes** → **Call _NHS Direct_**

No ↓

Self care advice

- Give your child regular Paracetamol (e.g. Calpol) to reduce the temperature (check the instructions on the packet for the right dose).
- Give them an extra amount of their favourite cool drink or ice lollies.
- Make sure your child is not over dressed – a vest and nappy/pants is enough clothing for them as long as the house is at the normal room temperature.
- Cover your child in a light cotton sheet when in bed.
- If condition gets worse or new symptoms develop, call _NHS Direct_.
- Make sure your child is up to date with all their immunisations.
- If you are still worried, call _NHS Direct_.

Before ringing _NHS Direct_ or **999**, it would be helpful if you think about the following and are ready to answer the questions if asked:
- How long they have been unwell
- If they are short of breath
- Their temperature (if possible)
- If there is a red/purple rash, light hurts their eyes, they are drowsy or bending the neck is painful
- If there is anyone else in the house with the same problem
- When they last had anything to drink or eat
- Any medicines they are taking at present.

We'll take the worry away

Fever in adults

You may have a fever, if you are feeling flushed, hot and sweaty (your temperature is over 38°C/100.4°F)

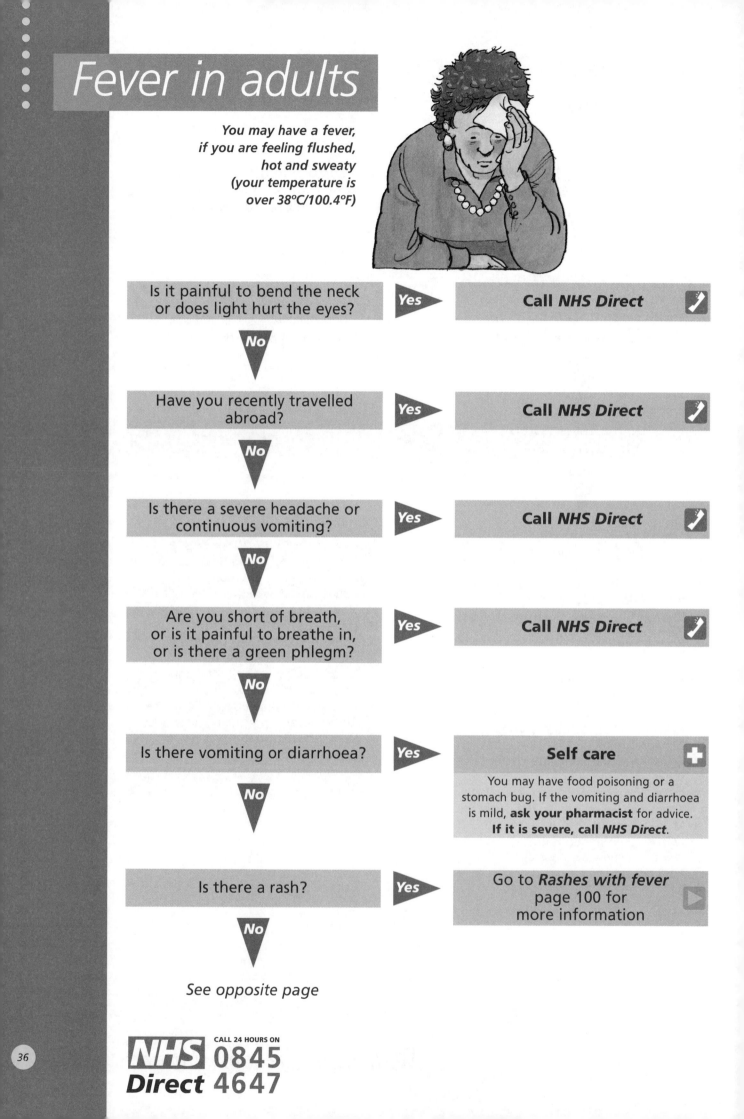

Is it painful to bend the neck or does light hurt the eyes?	**Yes** ▶	**Call NHS Direct**

No ▼

Have you recently travelled abroad?	**Yes** ▶	**Call NHS Direct**

No ▼

Is there a severe headache or continuous vomiting?	**Yes** ▶	**Call NHS Direct**

No ▼

Are you short of breath, or is it painful to breathe in, or is there a green phlegm?	**Yes** ▶	**Call NHS Direct**

No ▼

Is there vomiting or diarrhoea?	**Yes** ▶	**Self care**

You may have food poisoning or a stomach bug. If the vomiting and diarrhoea is mild, **ask your pharmacist** for advice. **If it is severe, call NHS Direct**.

No ▼

Is there a rash?	**Yes** ▶	Go to *Rashes with fever* page 100 for more information

No ▼

See opposite page

NHS Direct
CALL 24 HOURS ON
0845 4647

Is there a severe pain in your back?	**Yes** ▶	**Call *NHS Direct***

No ▼

Are there general aches and pains or a sore throat or a runny nose or sneezing?	**Yes** ▶	**Self care**

You probably have a viral infection such as a cold or flu. **Ask your pharmacist** for advice.

No ▼

Self care advice

- Try resting in bed if possible.
- Wear light clothing only.
- Take Paracetamol or Ibuprofen (follow the manufacturer's instructions) to help keep the temperature down.
- Increase your fluid intake.
- Make sure the room temperature is not too warm.
- If the condition gets worse or new symptoms develop, call **NHS Direct**.
- If you are still worried, call **NHS Direct**.

Before ringing *NHS Direct* or 999, it would be helpful if you think about the following and are ready to answer the questions if asked:
- How long you/they have been unwell
- If you/they have recently travelled abroad
- If there is a red/purple rash, light hurts the eyes or there is pain on bending the neck
- If you/they are very short of breath
- Your/their temperature (if possible)
- If there is anyone else in the house with the same problem
- When you/they last had anything to drink or eat
- Any medicines you/they are taking at present.

We'll take the worry away

Headache in children

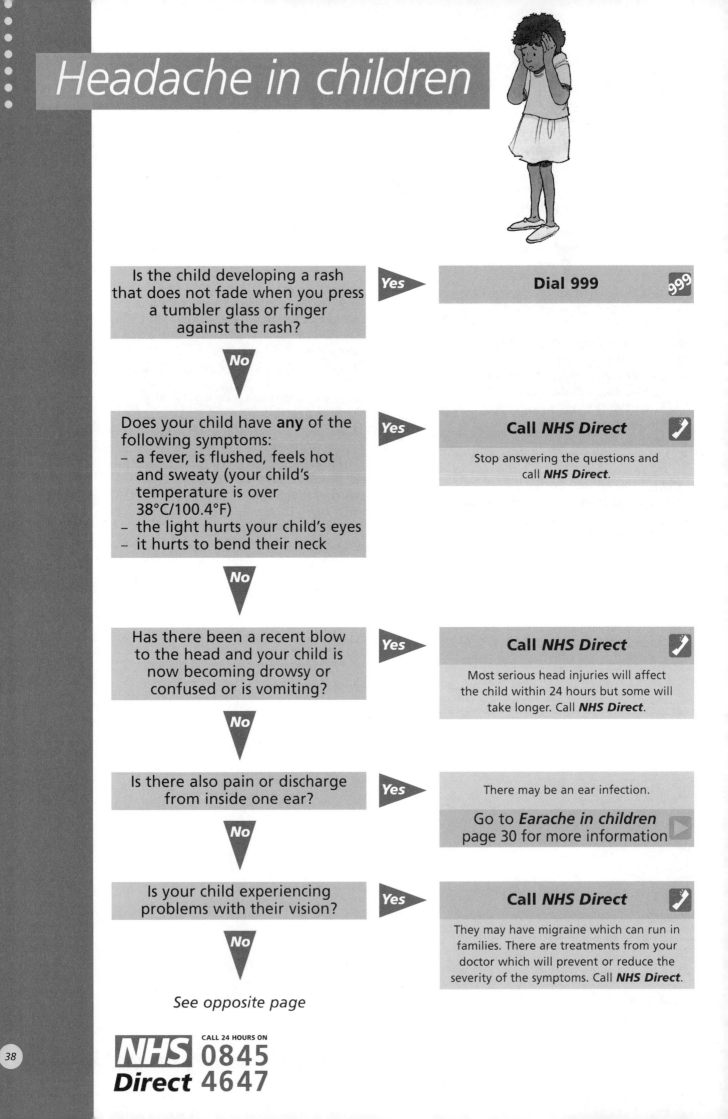

Is the child developing a rash that does not fade when you press a tumbler glass or finger against the rash?

Yes → **Dial 999** 999

No

Does your child have **any** of the following symptoms:
- a fever, is flushed, feels hot and sweaty (your child's temperature is over 38°C/100.4°F)
- the light hurts your child's eyes
- it hurts to bend their neck

Yes → **Call *NHS Direct***

Stop answering the questions and call ***NHS Direct***.

No

Has there been a recent blow to the head and your child is now becoming drowsy or confused or is vomiting?

Yes → **Call *NHS Direct***

Most serious head injuries will affect the child within 24 hours but some will take longer. Call ***NHS Direct***.

No

Is there also pain or discharge from inside one ear?

Yes → There may be an ear infection.

Go to *Earache in children* page 30 for more information

No

Is your child experiencing problems with their vision?

Yes → **Call *NHS Direct***

They may have migraine which can run in families. There are treatments from your doctor which will prevent or reduce the severity of the symptoms. Call ***NHS Direct***.

No

See opposite page

NHS Direct
CALL 24 HOURS ON
0845 4647

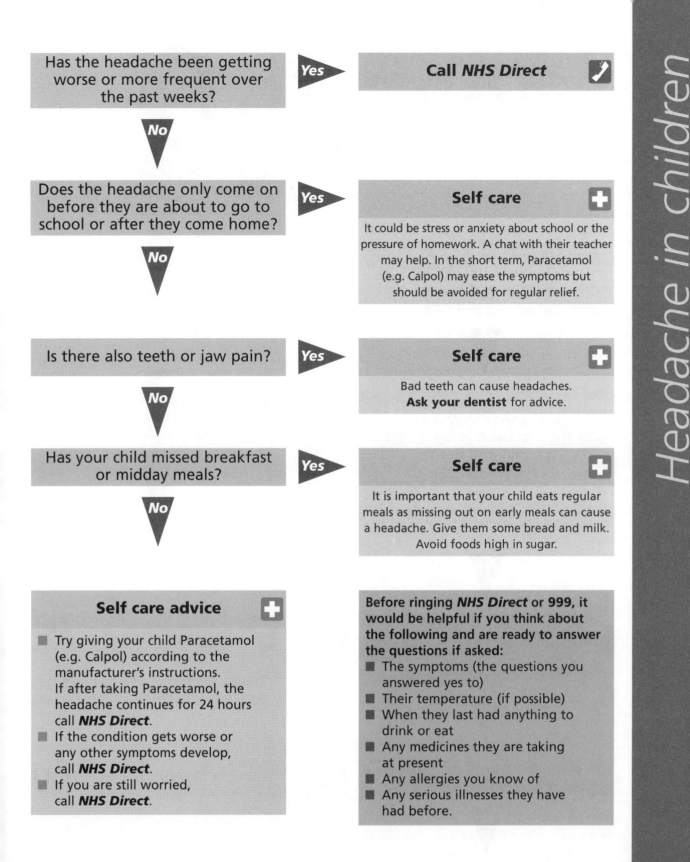

Has the headache been getting worse or more frequent over the past weeks?

Yes ▶ **Call *NHS Direct***

No ▼

Does the headache only come on before they are about to go to school or after they come home?

Yes ▶

Self care

It could be stress or anxiety about school or the pressure of homework. A chat with their teacher may help. In the short term, Paracetamol (e.g. Calpol) may ease the symptoms but should be avoided for regular relief.

No ▼

Is there also teeth or jaw pain?

Yes ▶

Self care

Bad teeth can cause headaches. **Ask your dentist** for advice.

No ▼

Has your child missed breakfast or midday meals?

Yes ▶

Self care

It is important that your child eats regular meals as missing out on early meals can cause a headache. Give them some bread and milk. Avoid foods high in sugar.

No ▼

Self care advice

- Try giving your child Paracetamol (e.g. Calpol) according to the manufacturer's instructions. If after taking Paracetamol, the headache continues for 24 hours call ***NHS Direct***.
- If the condition gets worse or any other symptoms develop, call ***NHS Direct***.
- If you are still worried, call ***NHS Direct***.

Before ringing ***NHS Direct*** or 999, it would be helpful if you think about the following and are ready to answer the questions if asked:
- The symptoms (the questions you answered yes to)
- Their temperature (if possible)
- When they last had anything to drink or eat
- Any medicines they are taking at present
- Any allergies you know of
- Any serious illnesses they have had before.

We'll take the worry away

Headache in adults

Is the person developing a rash that does not fade when you press a tumbler glass or finger against the rash?

Yes ▶ **Dial 999** 999

No

Do you have **any** of the following symptoms:
- Is there a fever, you are feeling flushed, hot and sweaty (your temperature is over 38°C/100.4°F)
- the light hurts your eyes
- it hurts to bend your neck?

Yes ▶ There is more advice in *Fever in adults* but if the pain is severe stop answering the questions and call *NHS Direct*.

Go to *Fever in adults* page 36 for more information ▶

No

Has there been a recent blow to the head and now the person is becoming drowsy or confused or is vomiting?

Yes ▶ **Dial 999** 999

Most serious head injuries will affect the person within 24 hours but some will take longer. **Dial 999**.

No

Is the pain behind one eye or is your vision affected?

Yes ▶ **Call *NHS Direct***

No

Are there visual patterns?

Yes ▶ **Self care** ✚

You may have a migraine. There are treatments from your pharmacist which will help or reduce the severity of the symptoms.

No

See opposite page

NHS Direct CALL 24 HOURS ON 0845 4647

Did the headache follow a time of excessive drinking?

Yes

No

Self care ✚

Hangover headaches can be severe but usually respond to plenty of fluids and Paracetamol. Your pharmacist will advise. For more information see *Hangovers* page 106.

Go to *Hangovers* page 106 for more information ▶

Is there any change in vision, hearing, taste or balance or is there increased vomiting?

Yes

No

Call *NHS Direct* ✎

Is your headache worse when bending forward?

Yes

No

Self care ✚

You may have sinusitis, an infection of the spaces in the bones of the face. Take strong painkillers according to the manufacturer's instructions and ring *NHS Direct*.

Is the headache worse during stress or anxiety such as while at work or during stressful times at home?

Yes

No

Self care ✚

It could be a stress headache which will respond well to either avoiding, or dealing with, those things causing the stress, or better coping methods such as relaxation techniques. Ask your practice nurse about relaxation techniques. Paracetamol will help in the short term but should be avoided for regular use.

Self care advice ✚

■ A common cause of early morning headaches is grinding your teeth at night. You should see your dentist.
■ Take regular painkillers such as Paracetamol, following the manufacturer's instructions for correct doses.
■ Wrapping a warm towel around the sufferer's neck may help relieve headaches caused through tension.
■ Sometimes a cold flannel placed on the area of the pain can be soothing.
■ If new symptoms develop, your headache gets worse or does not go away, call *NHS Direct*.
■ If you are still worried, call *NHS Direct*.

Before ringing *NHS Direct* or 999, it would be helpful if you think about the following and are ready to answer the questions if asked:
■ The symptoms (the questions you answered yes to)
■ Your/their temperature (if possible)
■ When you/they last had anything to drink or eat
■ Any medicines you/they are taking at present
■ Any allergies you know of
■ Any serious illnesses you/they have had before.

We'll take the worry away

Head injury in children

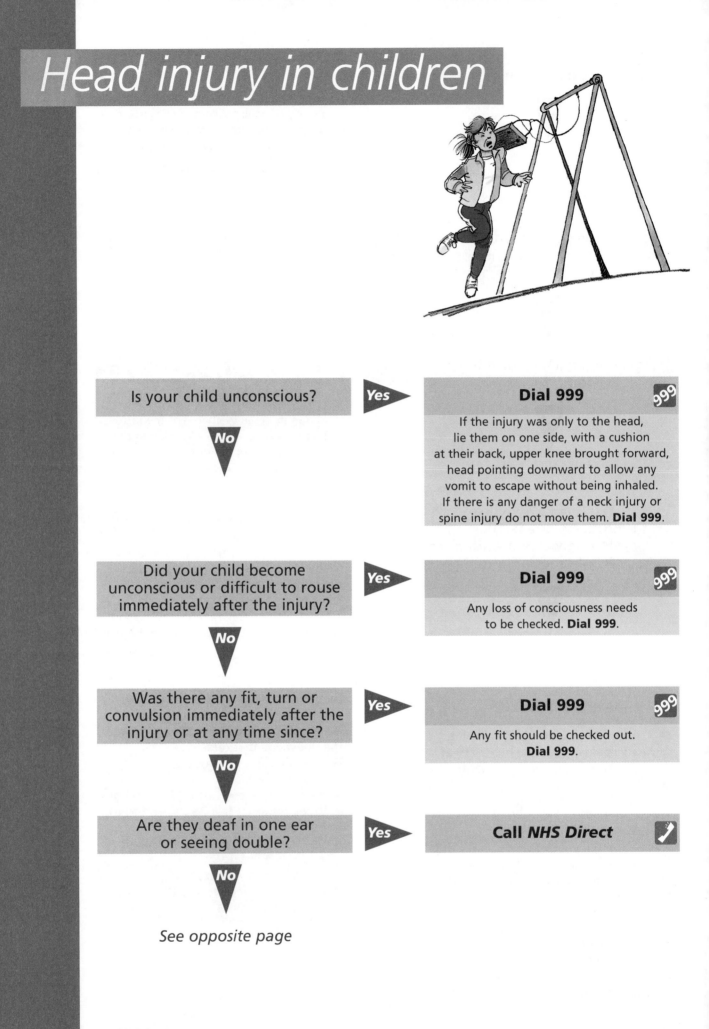

Is your child unconscious?

Yes → **Dial 999** `999`

If the injury was only to the head, lie them on one side, with a cushion at their back, upper knee brought forward, head pointing downward to allow any vomit to escape without being inhaled. If there is any danger of a neck injury or spine injury do not move them. **Dial 999**.

No ▼

Did your child become unconscious or difficult to rouse immediately after the injury?

Yes → **Dial 999** `999`

Any loss of consciousness needs to be checked. **Dial 999**.

No ▼

Was there any fit, turn or convulsion immediately after the injury or at any time since?

Yes → **Dial 999** `999`

Any fit should be checked out. **Dial 999**.

No ▼

Are they deaf in one ear or seeing double?

Yes → **Call *NHS Direct***

No ▼

See opposite page

NHS CALL 24 HOURS ON **0845**
Direct **4647**

Have they vomited more than twice since the accident?

Yes

Call NHS Direct

Head injuries do tend to make children vomit but the vomiting should stop soon afterwards. If the vomiting comes on later, or more than twice, call **NHS Direct**.

No

Are they increasingly difficult to rouse afterwards?

Yes

Call NHS Direct

Children do tend to sleep after a head injury. This is fine so long as you can rouse them every hour for the first six hours after the injury or they are not vomiting. Otherwise call **NHS Direct**.

No

Self care advice

- Place a cold facecloth over the bruised area.
- Give your child Paracetamol (e.g. Calpol) if you think they are in pain – read the instructions for the correct dose.
- Encourage your child to rest quietly for the next 48 hours and observe for signs of deterioration. This may include frequent bouts of sickness and abnormal behaviour. If there is any deterioration call **NHS Direct**.
- If your child's symptoms worsen or any new symptoms develop, call **NHS Direct**.
- If you are still worried, call **NHS Direct**.

Before ringing NHS Direct or 999, it would be helpful if you think about the following and are ready to answer the questions if asked:
- If they are unconscious or were knocked out for a while
- When the injury happened and how long they have been unwell
- If there is a problem with their vision, hearing or balance
- If they are vomiting, confused or very drowsy
- If there was any fit afterwards
- When they last had anything to drink or eat
- Any medicines they are taking at present.

We'll take the worry away

Poisoning

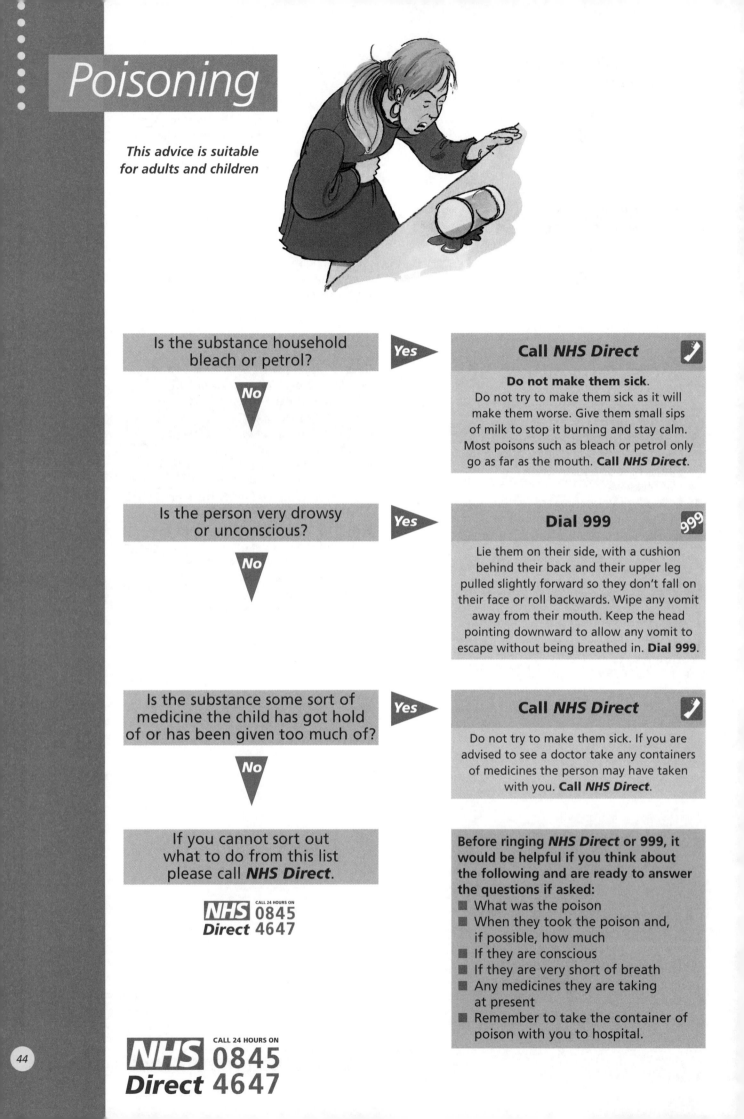

This advice is suitable for adults and children

Is the substance household bleach or petrol?

Yes ▶

Call *NHS Direct*

Do not make them sick.
Do not try to make them sick as it will make them worse. Give them small sips of milk to stop it burning and stay calm. Most poisons such as bleach or petrol only go as far as the mouth. **Call *NHS Direct***.

No ▼

Is the person very drowsy or unconscious?

Yes ▶

Dial 999

999

Lie them on their side, with a cushion behind their back and their upper leg pulled slightly forward so they don't fall on their face or roll backwards. Wipe any vomit away from their mouth. Keep the head pointing downward to allow any vomit to escape without being breathed in. **Dial 999**.

No ▼

Is the substance some sort of medicine the child has got hold of or has been given too much of?

Yes ▶

Call *NHS Direct*

Do not try to make them sick. If you are advised to see a doctor take any containers of medicines the person may have taken with you. **Call *NHS Direct***.

No ▼

If you cannot sort out what to do from this list please call *NHS Direct*.

NHS CALL 24 HOURS ON **0845**
Direct **4647**

Before ringing *NHS Direct* or 999, it would be helpful if you think about the following and are ready to answer the questions if asked:
- What was the poison
- When they took the poison and, if possible, how much
- If they are conscious
- If they are very short of breath
- Any medicines they are taking at present
- Remember to take the container of poison with you to hospital.

NHS CALL 24 HOURS ON **0845**
Direct **4647**

Self care advice

- Lock all chemicals and medicines away in a child-proof container.

- Keep all products in their original containers. Never put any medicines or chemicals such as weed-killer in soft drink bottles.

- Never refer to medicines as sweets.

- Clean out old medicines frequently and return them for safe destruction to your local community pharmacist.

- Rinse empty containers and throw them out in a safe place.

- Never take or give any medicines in the dark.

- Wherever possible buy products that have child resistant caps.

- Store cleaning products out of reach and where possible out of sight of children.

- Don't store medicines or cleaning agents near food.

- Keep the number of the local poisons unit, your family doctor and your local hospital ready to hand.

- Try taking a safety tour of your home with any young children and see if you can get them to point out the poisons.

- Ask the Royal Society for the Prevention of Accidents for advice on 0121 248 2000.

Below is a list of products that could be dangerous:

- Dish washing liquid
- Scouring soap
- Window cleaner
- Oven cleaner
- Medicines
- Vitamins
- Furniture polish
- Drain cleaner
- Ammonia
- Washing powder
- Bleach
- Fabric softener
- Dye

- Rat/ant poisons
- Moth balls

- Petrol
- Car wax/soaps
- Weedkiller/pesticides
- Paint
- Windscreen washer fluid
- Antifreeze

- Cosmetic products
- Shampoo
- Medications
- Cleansers
- Perfume
- Medicines/painkillers

We'll take the worry away

Sore throat in adults

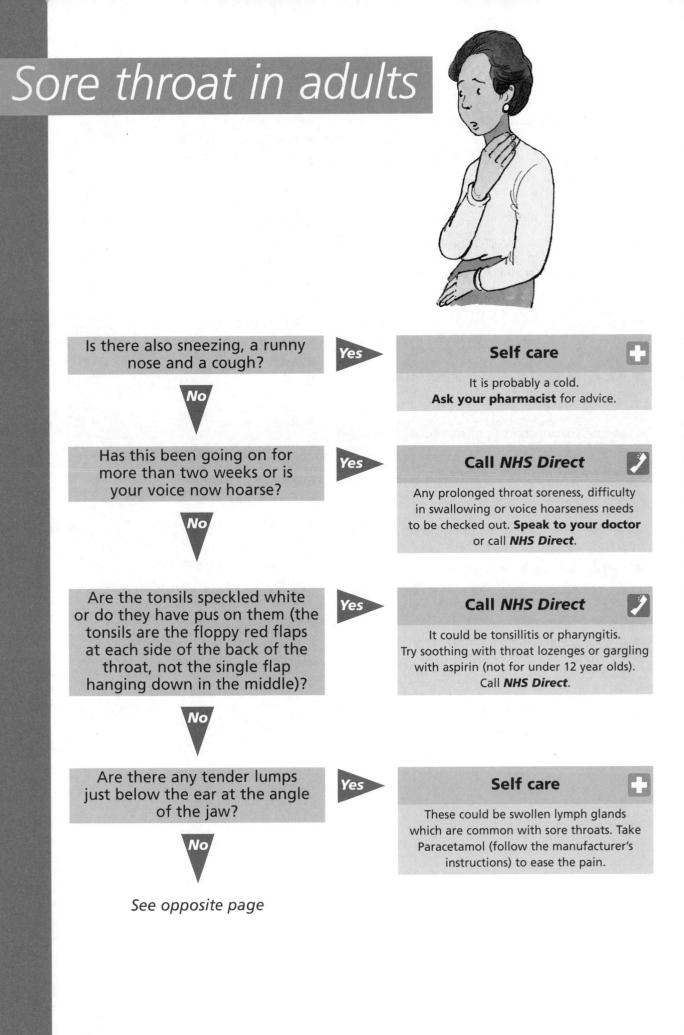

Is there also sneezing, a runny nose and a cough?

Yes →

Self care ✚

It is probably a cold.
Ask your pharmacist for advice.

No ▼

Has this been going on for more than two weeks or is your voice now hoarse?

Yes →

Call *NHS Direct*

Any prolonged throat soreness, difficulty in swallowing or voice hoarseness needs to be checked out. **Speak to your doctor** or call *NHS Direct*.

No ▼

Are the tonsils speckled white or do they have pus on them (the tonsils are the floppy red flaps at each side of the back of the throat, not the single flap hanging down in the middle)?

Yes →

Call *NHS Direct*

It could be tonsillitis or pharyngitis. Try soothing with throat lozenges or gargling with aspirin (not for under 12 year olds). Call *NHS Direct*.

No ▼

Are there any tender lumps just below the ear at the angle of the jaw?

Yes →

Self care ✚

These could be swollen lymph glands which are common with sore throats. Take Paracetamol (follow the manufacturer's instructions) to ease the pain.

No ▼

See opposite page

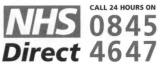

CALL 24 HOURS ON
NHS Direct 0845 4647

Is there a fever, are you feeling flushed, hot and sweaty (the temperature is over 38°C/100.4°F)?

Yes

Self care

If you also have a general feeling of being unwell, a cough and a headache you probably have a viral infection which will settle on its own. Take Paracetamol (follow the manufacturer's instructions).

No

Is it impossible to swallow your own saliva?

Yes

Call *NHS Direct*

If your throat is so swollen you need medical advice, call **NHS Direct**.

No

Self care advice

- Increase fluid intake, drink something non-alcoholic at least every hour.
- Take regular pain relief such as Paracetamol, following the manufacturer's instructions for correct dosage.
- Avoid foods that cause discomfort during swallowing.
- Throat remedies such as zinc lozenges from the pharmacist are available – they can advise you.
- If new symptoms develop or if your condition worsens, call **NHS Direct**.
- If you are still worried, call **NHS Direct**.

Before ringing **NHS Direct** or 999, it would be helpful if you think about the following and are ready to answer the questions if asked:
- How long you/they have been unwell
- If you/they are very short of breath or cannot swallow their own saliva
- Your/their temperature (if possible)
- Any medicines you/they are taking at present.

We'll take the worry away

Toothache

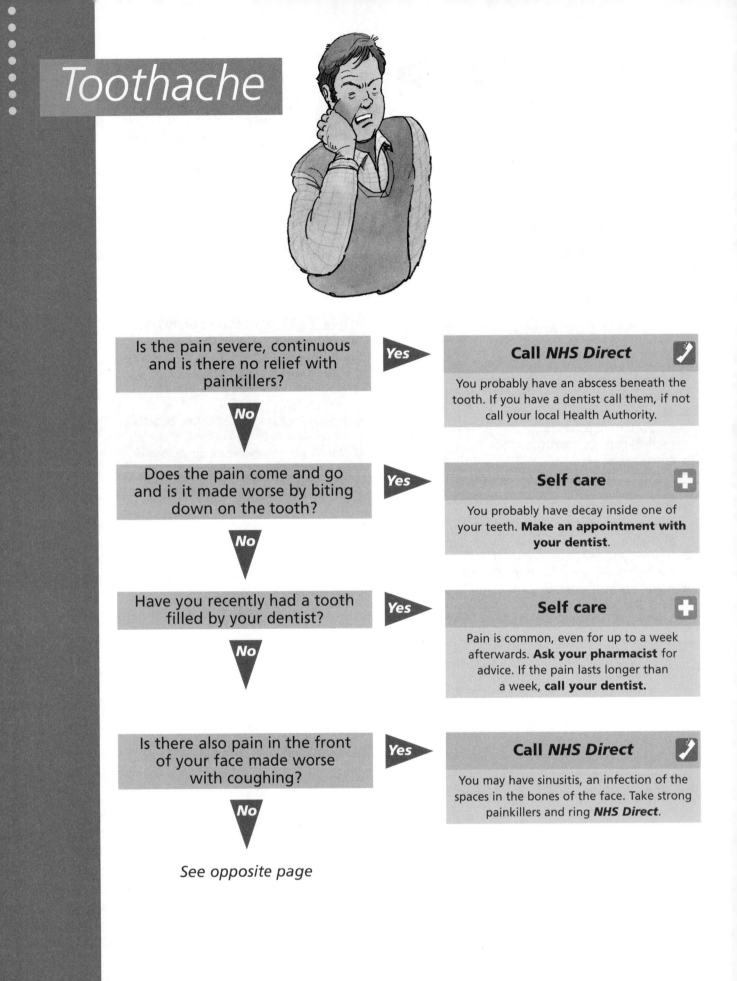

Is the pain severe, continuous and is there no relief with painkillers?

Yes → **Call NHS Direct**

You probably have an abscess beneath the tooth. If you have a dentist call them, if not call your local Health Authority.

No

Does the pain come and go and is it made worse by biting down on the tooth?

Yes → **Self care**

You probably have decay inside one of your teeth. **Make an appointment with your dentist**.

No

Have you recently had a tooth filled by your dentist?

Yes → **Self care**

Pain is common, even for up to a week afterwards. **Ask your pharmacist** for advice. If the pain lasts longer than a week, **call your dentist.**

No

Is there also pain in the front of your face made worse with coughing?

Yes → **Call NHS Direct**

You may have sinusitis, an infection of the spaces in the bones of the face. Take strong painkillers and ring **NHS Direct**.

No

See opposite page

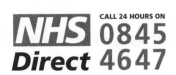

NHS Direct

CALL 24 HOURS ON
0845 4647

Is there a foul smell in your mouth?

Yes

No

Self care

Halitosis, smelly breath, can be caused by a number of things, not least food or drink but a tooth abscess is a common cause. Avoid over use of breath fresheners or antiseptic mouthwashes. **See your dentist.**

Self care advice

- Take maximum dose of painkillers such as Paracetamol or Ibuprofen according to the manufacturer's instructions.
- Avoid drinks that are too hot or too cold until your dentist has examined your teeth.
- Avoid food/drinks containing sugar.
- Contact your dentist at the first available opportunity.
- If you don't have a dentist call your local Health Authority or **NHS Direct** who will be able to help.
- If you are still worried, call **NHS Direct**.

We'll take the worry away

Vomiting in babies

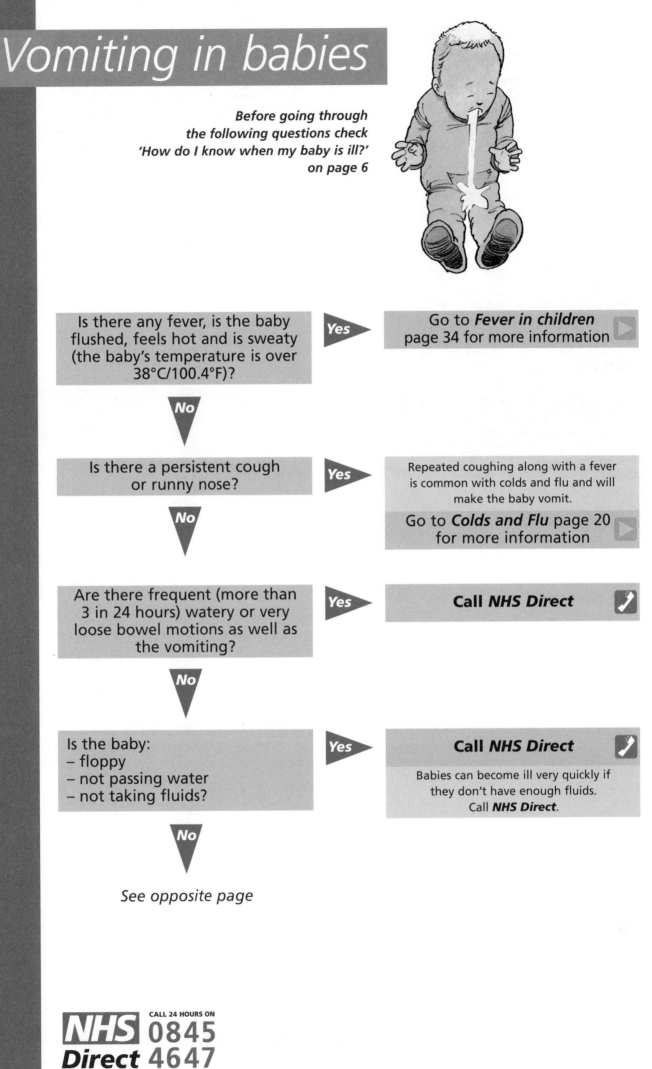

*Before going through
the following questions check
'How do I know when my baby is ill?'
on page 6*

Is there any fever, is the baby flushed, feels hot and is sweaty (the baby's temperature is over 38°C/100.4°F)?

Yes ▶ Go to *Fever in children* page 34 for more information ▷

No ▼

Is there a persistent cough or runny nose?

Yes ▶ Repeated coughing along with a fever is common with colds and flu and will make the baby vomit.

Go to *Colds and Flu* page 20 for more information ▷

No ▼

Are there frequent (more than 3 in 24 hours) watery or very loose bowel motions as well as the vomiting?

Yes ▶ **Call *NHS Direct***

No ▼

**Is the baby:
– floppy
– not passing water
– not taking fluids?**

Yes ▶ **Call *NHS Direct***

Babies can become ill very quickly if they don't have enough fluids.
Call *NHS Direct*.

No ▼

See opposite page

NHS Direct

CALL 24 HOURS ON
0845 4647

Is the vomiting forceful (projectile) and after each feed or is there weight loss?

Yes ▶

Call *NHS Direct*

There may be a problem with the emptying of the stomach. Call *NHS Direct*.

No ▼

Is the vomiting just small amounts after feeds and the baby is otherwise fine?

Yes ▶

Self care ➕

Babies often bring up small amounts of their feed but it should look similar to their milk feed and not come out with any force. Winding helps. Using an over large hole in the teat when bottle feeding is a common cause. Avoid over use of 'colic treatments'.

No ▼

Is the baby crying continuously or obviously in pain?

Yes ▶

Call *NHS Direct*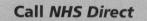

It can be difficult to tell when a baby is in severe pain as well as vomiting. A change in the way the baby is crying, particularly when previously well, or if there is a rash or fever, call *NHS Direct*.

No ▼

Self care advice ➕

- If breast-feeding, continue as normal, unless vomiting has occurred more than twice, in which case call *NHS Direct*.
- If bottle-feeding, introduce rehydration fluids (e.g. Dioralyte) in small quantities as per the manufacturer's instructions on the package. Speak to your pharmacist.
- Do not give large amounts of fluids in one go and reintroduce milk gradually.
- If the condition has not improved within 2 hours or the baby does not have a wet nappy or other symptoms have developed, call *NHS Direct*.
- If you are still worried, call *NHS Direct*.

Before ringing *NHS Direct* or 999, it would be helpful if you think about the following and are ready to answer the questions if asked:
- The symptoms (the questions you answered yes to)
- Their temperature (if possible)
- When they last had anything to drink or eat
- Any medicines they are taking at present
- Any allergies you know of
- Any serious illnesses they have had before.

We'll take the worry away

Vomiting in children

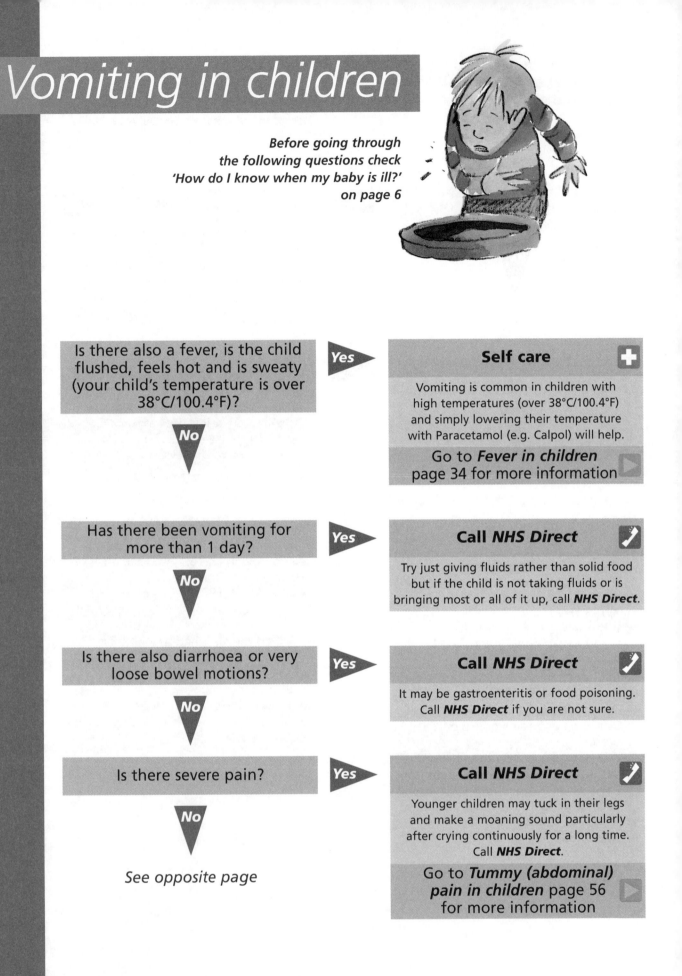

*Before going through
the following questions check
'How do I know when my baby is ill?'
on page 6*

Is there also a fever, is the child flushed, feels hot and is sweaty (your child's temperature is over 38°C/100.4°F)?

Yes → **Self care** ✚

Vomiting is common in children with high temperatures (over 38°C/100.4°F) and simply lowering their temperature with Paracetamol (e.g. Calpol) will help.

Go to *Fever in children* page 34 for more information ▶

No ▼

Has there been vomiting for more than 1 day?

Yes → **Call *NHS Direct*** 🖊

Try just giving fluids rather than solid food but if the child is not taking fluids or is bringing most or all of it up, call ***NHS Direct***.

No ▼

Is there also diarrhoea or very loose bowel motions?

Yes → **Call *NHS Direct*** 🖊

It may be gastroenteritis or food poisoning. Call ***NHS Direct*** if you are not sure.

No ▼

Is there severe pain?

Yes → **Call *NHS Direct*** 🖊

Younger children may tuck in their legs and make a moaning sound particularly after crying continuously for a long time. Call ***NHS Direct***.

Go to *Tummy (abdominal) pain in children* page 56 for more information ▶

No ▼

See opposite page

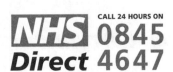

NHS Direct

CALL 24 HOURS ON
0845 4647

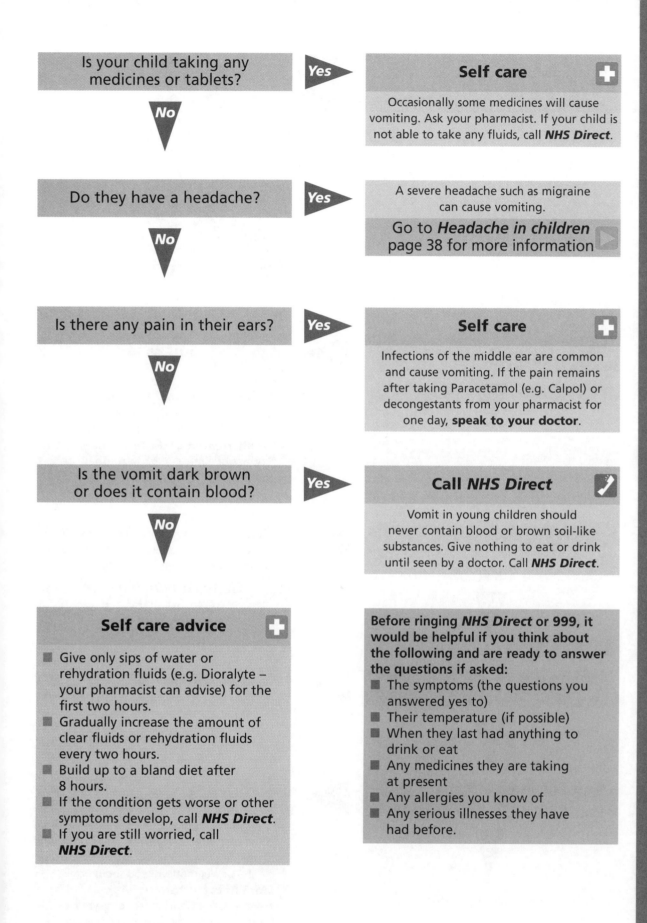

Is your child taking any medicines or tablets?

Yes

No

Self care ✚

Occasionally some medicines will cause vomiting. Ask your pharmacist. If your child is not able to take any fluids, call **NHS Direct**.

Do they have a headache?

Yes

No

A severe headache such as migraine can cause vomiting.

Go to *Headache in children* page 38 for more information ▶

Is there any pain in their ears?

Yes

No

Self care ✚

Infections of the middle ear are common and cause vomiting. If the pain remains after taking Paracetamol (e.g. Calpol) or decongestants from your pharmacist for one day, **speak to your doctor**.

Is the vomit dark brown or does it contain blood?

Yes

No

Call *NHS Direct* ✐

Vomit in young children should never contain blood or brown soil-like substances. Give nothing to eat or drink until seen by a doctor. Call **NHS Direct**.

Self care advice ✚

- Give only sips of water or rehydration fluids (e.g. Dioralyte – your pharmacist can advise) for the first two hours.
- Gradually increase the amount of clear fluids or rehydration fluids every two hours.
- Build up to a bland diet after 8 hours.
- If the condition gets worse or other symptoms develop, call **NHS Direct**.
- If you are still worried, call **NHS Direct**.

Before ringing *NHS Direct* or 999, it would be helpful if you think about the following and are ready to answer the questions if asked:
- The symptoms (the questions you answered yes to)
- Their temperature (if possible)
- When they last had anything to drink or eat
- Any medicines they are taking at present
- Any allergies you know of
- Any serious illnesses they have had before.

We'll take the worry away

Vomiting in adults

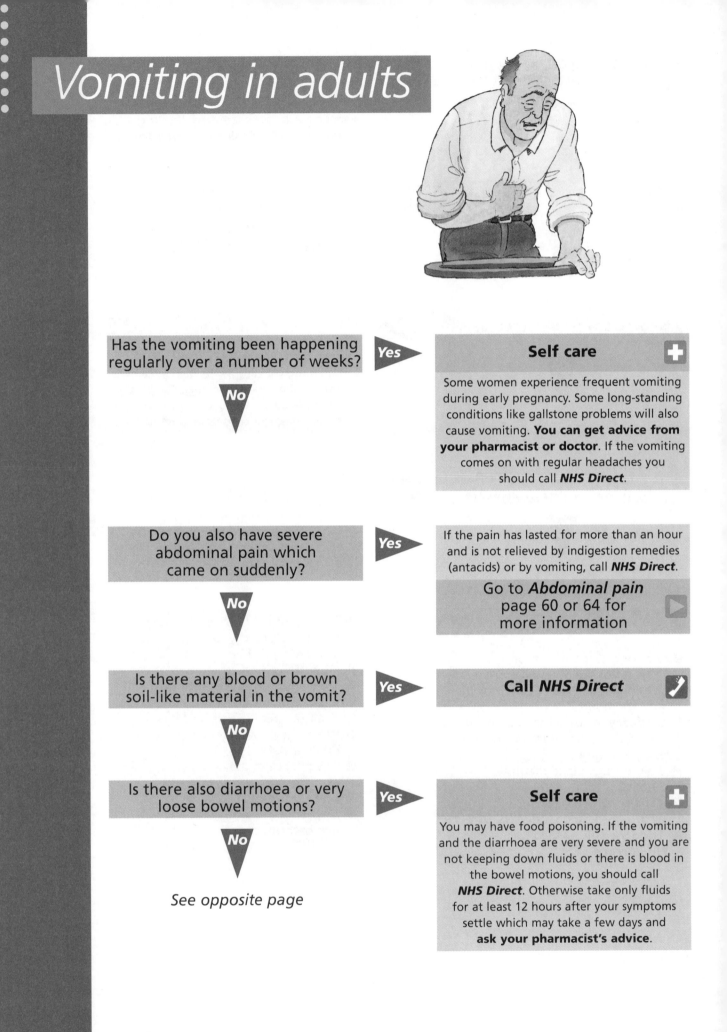

Has the vomiting been happening regularly over a number of weeks?

Yes

No

Self care ➕

Some women experience frequent vomiting during early pregnancy. Some long-standing conditions like gallstone problems will also cause vomiting. **You can get advice from your pharmacist or doctor**. If the vomiting comes on with regular headaches you should call **NHS Direct**.

Do you also have severe abdominal pain which came on suddenly?

Yes

No

If the pain has lasted for more than an hour and is not relieved by indigestion remedies (antacids) or by vomiting, call **NHS Direct**.

Go to **Abdominal pain** page 60 or 64 for more information ▷

Is there any blood or brown soil-like material in the vomit?

Yes

No

Call **NHS Direct** 🔦

Is there also diarrhoea or very loose bowel motions?

Yes

No

See opposite page

Self care ➕

You may have food poisoning. If the vomiting and the diarrhoea are very severe and you are not keeping down fluids or there is blood in the bowel motions, you should call **NHS Direct**. Otherwise take only fluids for at least 12 hours after your symptoms settle which may take a few days and **ask your pharmacist's advice**.

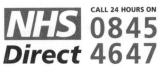

NHS Direct

CALL 24 HOURS ON
0845 4647

Do you have a severe headache? **Yes**

No

Dial 999

Any severe pain will cause vomiting but if you do not normally suffer from headaches such as migraine, or there has been a recent head injury, or the light is hurting your eyes, you should **dial 999**.

Self care advice ✚

- Try small amounts of clear fluids or rehydration fluids (e.g. Dioralyte) from your pharmacist.
- Build up the amount of fluids from sips to a cup full over the next 12 hours.
- 12 hours after the last bout of vomiting, introduce bland foods back into your diet (this includes dry biscuits, toast or crackers).
- Avoid milk in your diet during this period.
- Sometimes the cause of vomiting can be bacterial infection, and can be spread to other people.
- It is therefore important to thoroughly clean all areas that have been in contact with the vomit.
- Be extra careful about personal hygiene, washing hands, etc.
- If the condition worsens or new symptoms develop, call **NHS Direct**.
- If you are still worried, call **NHS Direct**.

Before ringing *NHS Direct* or 999, it would be helpful if you think about the following and are ready to answer the questions if asked:
- The symptoms (the questions you answered yes to)
- Your/their temperature (if possible)
- When you/they last had anything to drink or eat
- Any medicines you/they are taking at present
- Any allergies you know of
- Any serious illnesses you/they have had before.

We'll take the worry away

Tummy (abdominal) pain in children

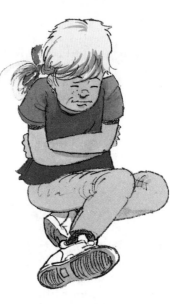

*Before going through
the following questions check
'How do I know when my baby is ill?'
on page 6*

Has your child just eaten a large amount of fruit or foods they do not usually eat?

Yes ▶

Self care ✚

Overeating, especially of acid fruit can cause tummy pain. Try simple indigestion remedies like milk. If the symptoms don't improve or they worsen or there are any other symptoms within 24 hours, call **NHS Direct**.

No ▼

Is your child constipated?

Yes ▶

Self care ✚

Not enough fluids, particularly in hot weather, can cause constipation in children. If the symptoms don't improve or if they develop a new symptom such as vomiting, call **NHS Direct**. Otherwise **ask your pharmacist** for advice.

No ▼

Does the tummy pain only come on before they are about to go to school or after they come home?

Yes ▶

Self care ✚

It could be stress or anxiety about school or the pressure of homework. A chat about it with their teacher may help. In the short term, Paracetamol (e.g. Calpol) may ease the symptoms but should be avoided for regular relief.

No ▼

If the child is male, is there a severe pain in one of his testicles which came on very suddenly?

Yes ▶

Call **NHS Direct** 🔦

No ▼

See opposite page

NHS CALL 24 HOURS ON
Direct **0845 4647**

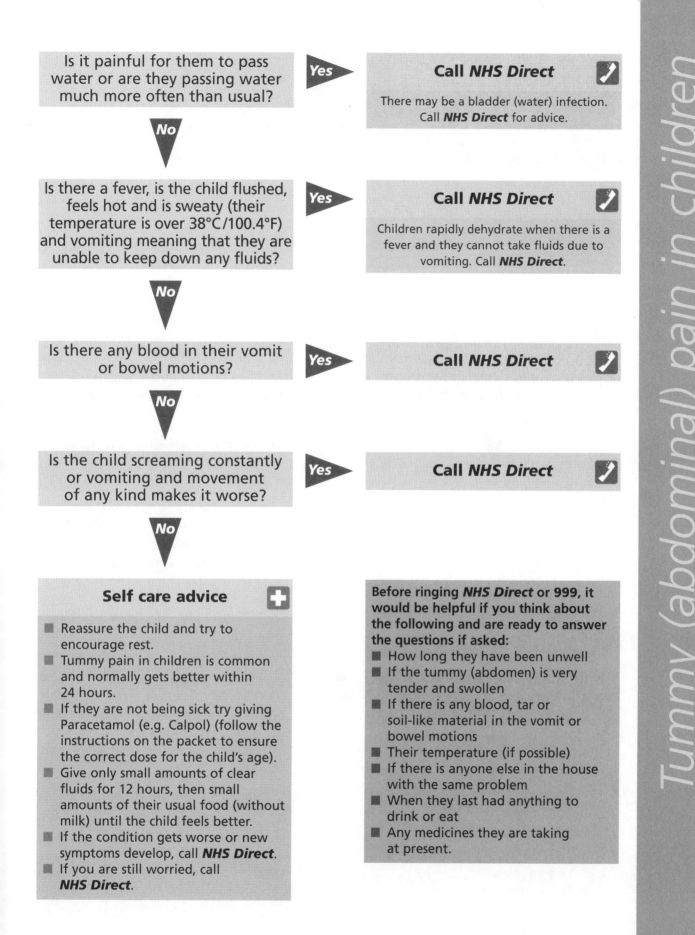

Is it painful for them to pass water or are they passing water much more often than usual?

Yes → **Call _NHS Direct_**

There may be a bladder (water) infection. Call **_NHS Direct_** for advice.

No

Is there a fever, is the child flushed, feels hot and is sweaty (their temperature is over 38°C/100.4°F) and vomiting meaning that they are unable to keep down any fluids?

Yes → **Call _NHS Direct_**

Children rapidly dehydrate when there is a fever and they cannot take fluids due to vomiting. Call **_NHS Direct_**.

No

Is there any blood in their vomit or bowel motions?

Yes → **Call _NHS Direct_**

No

Is the child screaming constantly or vomiting and movement of any kind makes it worse?

Yes → **Call _NHS Direct_**

No

Self care advice

- Reassure the child and try to encourage rest.
- Tummy pain in children is common and normally gets better within 24 hours.
- If they are not being sick try giving Paracetamol (e.g. Calpol) (follow the instructions on the packet to ensure the correct dose for the child's age).
- Give only small amounts of clear fluids for 12 hours, then small amounts of their usual food (without milk) until the child feels better.
- If the condition gets worse or new symptoms develop, call **_NHS Direct_**.
- If you are still worried, call **_NHS Direct_**.

Before ringing _NHS Direct_ or 999, it would be helpful if you think about the following and are ready to answer the questions if asked:

- How long they have been unwell
- If the tummy (abdomen) is very tender and swollen
- If there is any blood, tar or soil-like material in the vomit or bowel motions
- Their temperature (if possible)
- If there is anyone else in the house with the same problem
- When they last had anything to drink or eat
- Any medicines they are taking at present.

We'll take the worry away

Long-standing abdominal pain in adults

Is the pain a burning sensation deep inside the upper tummy, made worse when lying down or bending over?

Yes ▶

No

Self care ✚

You may have stomach acid leaking into the gullet which is common and is treatable with indigestion remedies (antacids) or medicines which block the production of stomach acid or make the stomach move its contents on quicker. You should use an extra pillow at night and avoid foods that bring on the pain. **Ask your pharmacist** for advice.
If the pain is severe or your bowel motions are tar-like black, you should call **NHS Direct**.

Go to **Hiatus hernia** page 107 for more information ▶

Is the pain relieved by drinking milk or taking indigestion remedies (antacids)?

Yes ▶

No

See opposite page

Self care ✚

Inflammation of the stomach wall (gastritis) is quite common, particularly after rich food or alcohol. It should settle with simple indigestion remedies. **Ask your pharmacist** for advice.
If the pain is severe or you are passing tar-like black bowel motions or are vomiting soil-like material, call **NHS Direct**.

Go to **Indigestion** page 109 and **Peptic ulcers** page 116 for more information ▶

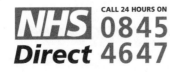
NHS Direct CALL 24 HOURS ON **0845 4647**

Is the pain on the right side just under the ribs and is your temperature raised?

 Yes

Self care

Avoid those foods, usually fatty meals, which trigger the pain. Take Paracetamol for the pain, avoid all food and drink only water until the pain subsides. If the problem continues you may become jaundiced with a yellow tinge to your skin and the whites of your eyes; **in these circumstances you should call *NHS Direct*.** If you have not been diagnosed as having gall stone problems by your doctor you should make an appointment.

 No

Is your appetite poor or have you lost weight over the past two months for no apparent reason?

 Yes

Call *NHS Direct*

If the symptoms are not getting better with indigestion remedies, call ***NHS Direct***.

 No

Do you get tummy bloating and have irregular bowel motions?

 Yes

Self care

You may have irritable bowel syndrome (IBS) which is common but not serious. Avoiding those things which make it worse, such as certain foods, stress etc, is important.
You should see your doctor if:
– the home treatment doesn't work after two weeks
– you pass blood in your motions
– your bowel motions are very dark black or covered with mucus
– there is an unexplained weight loss

Go to *Irritable bowel syndrome* page 110 for more information

No

Self care advice

- Try resting.
- If you are not vomiting, take fluids in small quantities only for the next 12 hours.
- Take simple painkillers such as Paracetamol (do not take aspirin or codeine).
- If the condition gets worse or other symptoms develop, call ***NHS Direct***.
- If you are still worried, call ***NHS Direct***.

We'll take the worry away

Female abdominal pain in adults

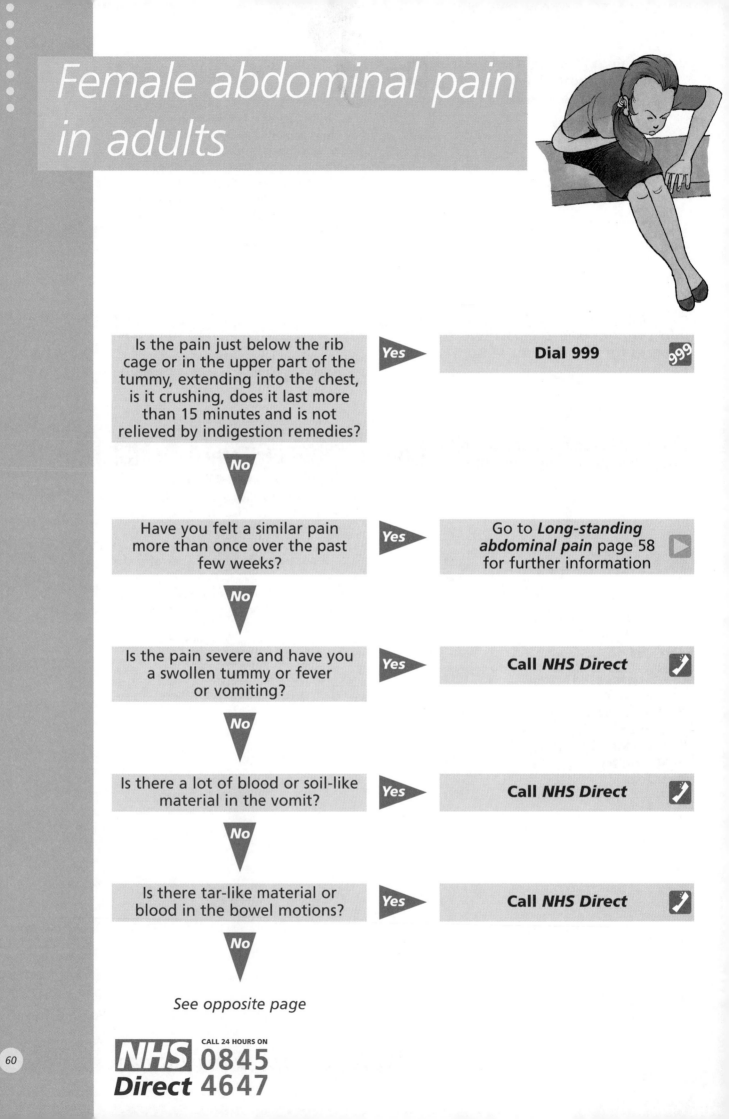

Is the pain just below the rib cage or in the upper part of the tummy, extending into the chest, is it crushing, does it last more than 15 minutes and is not relieved by indigestion remedies?

Yes → **Dial 999** 999

No ↓

Have you felt a similar pain more than once over the past few weeks?

Yes → Go to *Long-standing abdominal pain* page 58 for further information

No ↓

Is the pain severe and have you a swollen tummy or fever or vomiting?

Yes → **Call *NHS Direct***

No ↓

Is there a lot of blood or soil-like material in the vomit?

Yes → **Call *NHS Direct***

No ↓

Is there tar-like material or blood in the bowel motions?

Yes → **Call *NHS Direct***

No ↓

See opposite page

NHS
Direct
CALL 24 HOURS ON
0845 4647

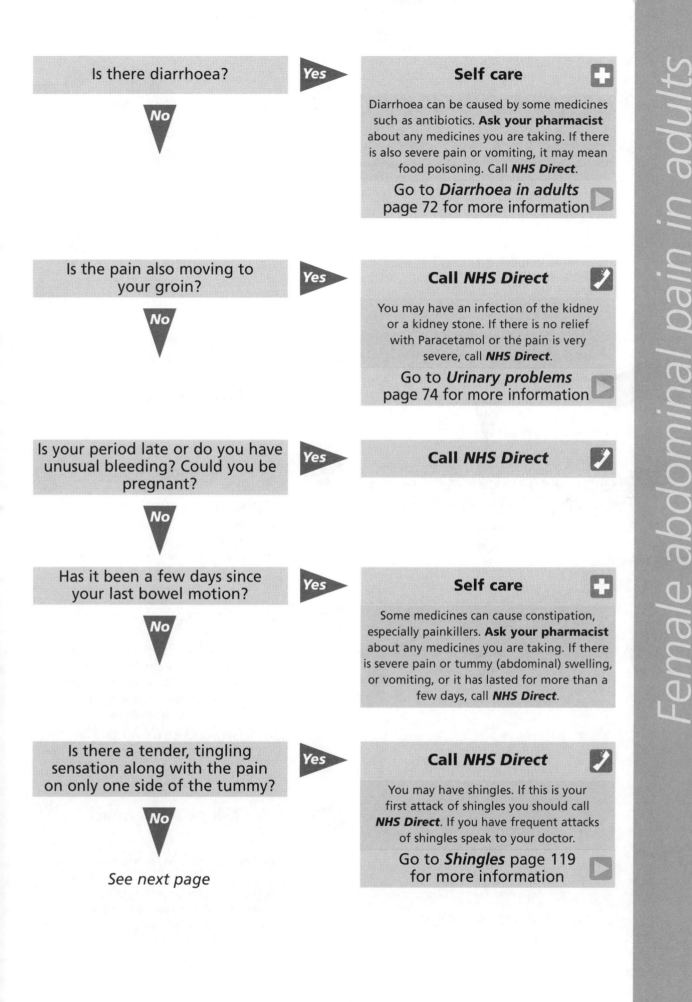

Is there diarrhoea?

Yes

No

Self care

Diarrhoea can be caused by some medicines such as antibiotics. **Ask your pharmacist** about any medicines you are taking. If there is also severe pain or vomiting, it may mean food poisoning. Call **NHS Direct**.

Go to *Diarrhoea in adults* page 72 for more information

Is the pain also moving to your groin?

Yes

No

Call *NHS Direct*

You may have an infection of the kidney or a kidney stone. If there is no relief with Paracetamol or the pain is very severe, call **NHS Direct**.

Go to *Urinary problems* page 74 for more information

Is your period late or do you have unusual bleeding? Could you be pregnant?

Yes

No

Call *NHS Direct*

Has it been a few days since your last bowel motion?

Yes

No

Self care

Some medicines can cause constipation, especially painkillers. **Ask your pharmacist** about any medicines you are taking. If there is severe pain or tummy (abdominal) swelling, or vomiting, or it has lasted for more than a few days, call **NHS Direct**.

Is there a tender, tingling sensation along with the pain on only one side of the tummy?

Yes

No

See next page

Call *NHS Direct*

You may have shingles. If this is your first attack of shingles you should call **NHS Direct**. If you have frequent attacks of shingles speak to your doctor.

Go to *Shingles* page 119 for more information

We'll take the worry away

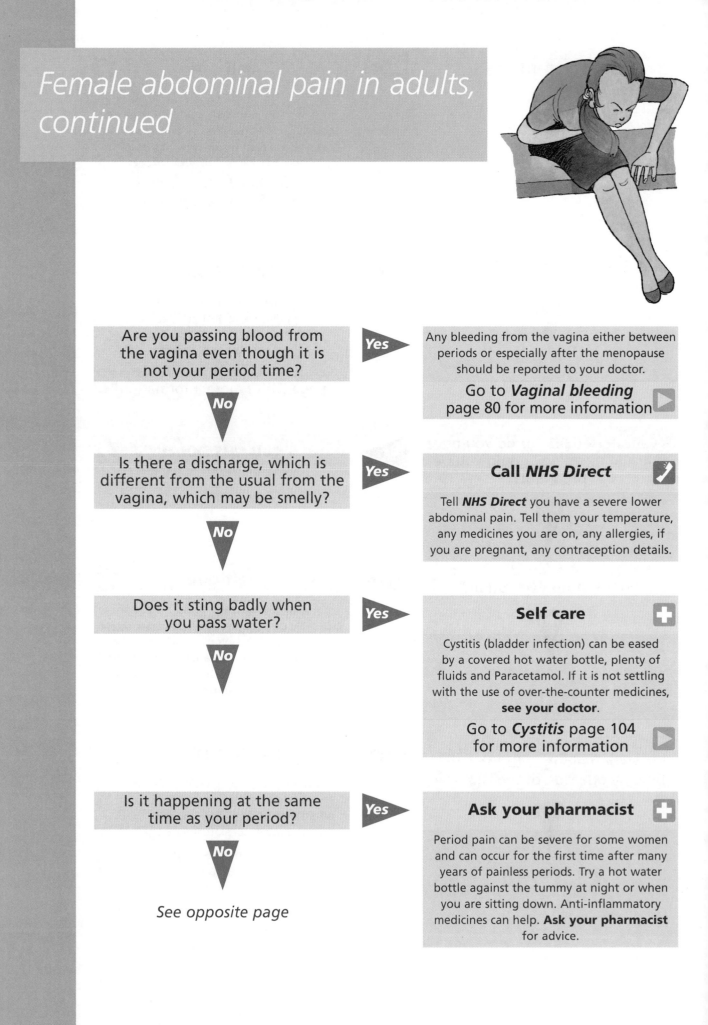

Are you passing blood from the vagina even though it is not your period time?

Yes → Any bleeding from the vagina either between periods or especially after the menopause should be reported to your doctor.

Go to *Vaginal bleeding* page 80 for more information

No ↓

Is there a discharge, which is different from the usual from the vagina, which may be smelly?

Yes → **Call *NHS Direct***

Tell ***NHS Direct*** you have a severe lower abdominal pain. Tell them your temperature, any medicines you are on, any allergies, if you are pregnant, any contraception details.

No ↓

Does it sting badly when you pass water?

Yes → **Self care**

Cystitis (bladder infection) can be eased by a covered hot water bottle, plenty of fluids and Paracetamol. If it is not settling with the use of over-the-counter medicines, **see your doctor**.

Go to *Cystitis* page 104 for more information

No ↓

Is it happening at the same time as your period?

Yes → **Ask your pharmacist**

Period pain can be severe for some women and can occur for the first time after many years of painless periods. Try a hot water bottle against the tummy at night or when you are sitting down. Anti-inflammatory medicines can help. **Ask your pharmacist** for advice.

No ↓

See opposite page

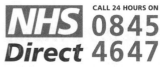

NHS Direct

CALL 24 HOURS ON
0845 4647

Self care advice

- Try to relieve the pain by resting.
- If you are not vomiting, try taking simple painkillers.
- If the condition gets worse or new symptoms develop, call **NHS Direct**.
- If you are still worried, call **NHS Direct**.

Before ringing *NHS Direct* or 999, it would be helpful if you think about the following and are ready to answer the questions if asked:

- How long you/they have been unwell
- If it may be a heart attack
- If you/they are pregnant
- If there is any vaginal bleeding
- If the tummy (abdomen) is very tender and distended
- If there is any blood, tar or soil-like material in the vomit or bowel motions
- If the pain is in the back moving down to the groin
- Your/their temperature (if possible)
- If there is anyone else in the house with the same problem
- When you/they last had anything to drink or eat
- Any medicines you/they are taking at present
- Any illnesses such as bowel, heart, stomach or kidney problems you/they have had before.

We'll take the worry away

Male abdominal pain in adults

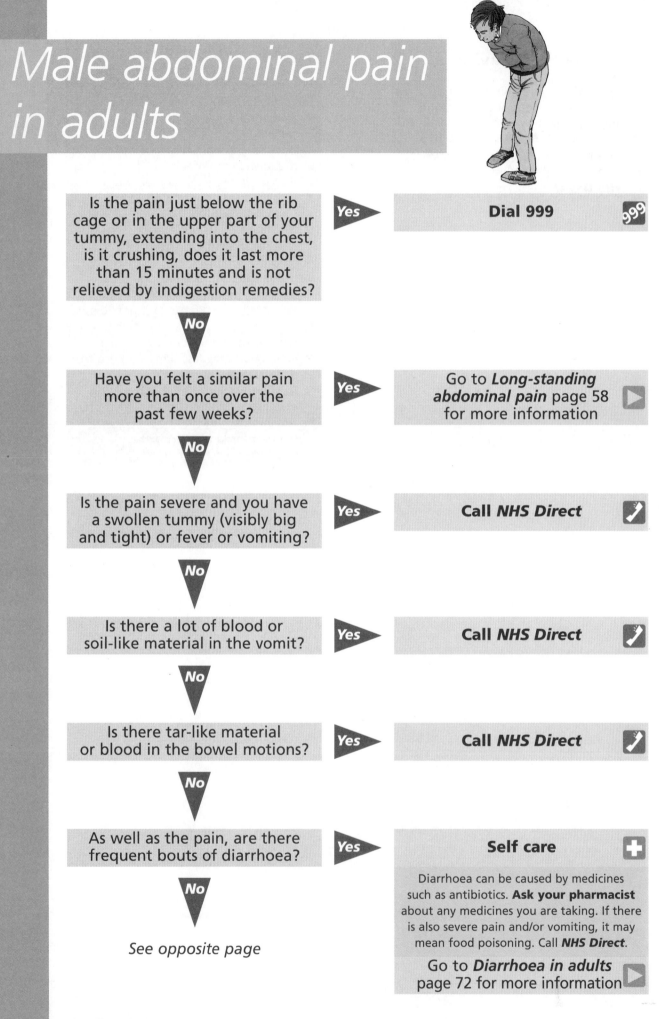

Is the pain just below the rib cage or in the upper part of your tummy, extending into the chest, is it crushing, does it last more than 15 minutes and is not relieved by indigestion remedies?

Yes → **Dial 999** `999`

No

Have you felt a similar pain more than once over the past few weeks?

Yes → Go to *Long-standing abdominal pain* page 58 for more information ▷

No

Is the pain severe and you have a swollen tummy (visibly big and tight) or fever or vomiting?

Yes → **Call *NHS Direct***

No

Is there a lot of blood or soil-like material in the vomit?

Yes → **Call *NHS Direct***

No

Is there tar-like material or blood in the bowel motions?

Yes → **Call *NHS Direct***

No

As well as the pain, are there frequent bouts of diarrhoea?

Yes → **Self care** ✚

Diarrhoea can be caused by medicines such as antibiotics. **Ask your pharmacist** about any medicines you are taking. If there is also severe pain and/or vomiting, it may mean food poisoning. Call ***NHS Direct***.

Go to *Diarrhoea in adults* page 72 for more information ▷

No

See opposite page

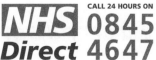

NHS Direct CALL 24 HOURS ON **0845 4647**

Is the pain also moving
to your groin?

Yes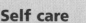

Self care

You may have an infection of the kidney
or a kidney stone. If there is no relief
with Paracetamol or the pain is very
severe, call **NHS Direct**.

Go to *Urinary problems*
page 76 for more information

No

Has it been a few days since your
last bowel motion?

Yes

Self care

Some medicines, especially painkillers, will
cause constipation. **Ask your pharmacist**
about any medicines you are taking. If there
is severe pain or tummy (abdominal) swelling,
or vomiting, or it has lasted for more than a
few days, **speak to your doctor**.

No

Is there a severe pain in one of
your testicles which came on
very suddenly?

Yes

Call *NHS Direct*

No

Is there a tender, tingling
sensation along with the pain on
only one side of the tummy?

Yes

Call *NHS Direct*

You may have shingles. If this is your first
attack of shingles you should call **NHS Direct**.
If you are having repeated attacks of shingles
you should **tell your doctor**.

Go to *Shingles* page 119
for more information

No

Self care advice

- Try to relieve the pain by resting.
- If you are not vomiting, try taking
  simple painkillers.
- Watch closely for signs of restlessness
  or the condition becoming worse –
  in which case call **NHS Direct**.
- If new symptoms develop or the pain
  gets worse, call **NHS Direct**.
- If you are still worried, call
  NHS Direct.

**Before ringing *NHS Direct* or 999, it
would be helpful if you think about
the following and are ready to answer
the questions if asked:**
- How long you/they have been unwell
- If it may be a heart attack
- If the tummy (abdomen) is very tender
  and swollen
- If there is any blood, tar or soil-like
  material in the vomit or bowel motions
- If the pain is in the back moving down
  the groin
- Your/their temperature (if possible),
- If there is anyone else in the house
  with the same problem
- When you/they last had anything to
  drink or eat
- Any medicines you/they are taking
  at present
- Any illnesses such as bowel, heart,
  stomach or kidney problems you/they
  have had before.

Backache in adults

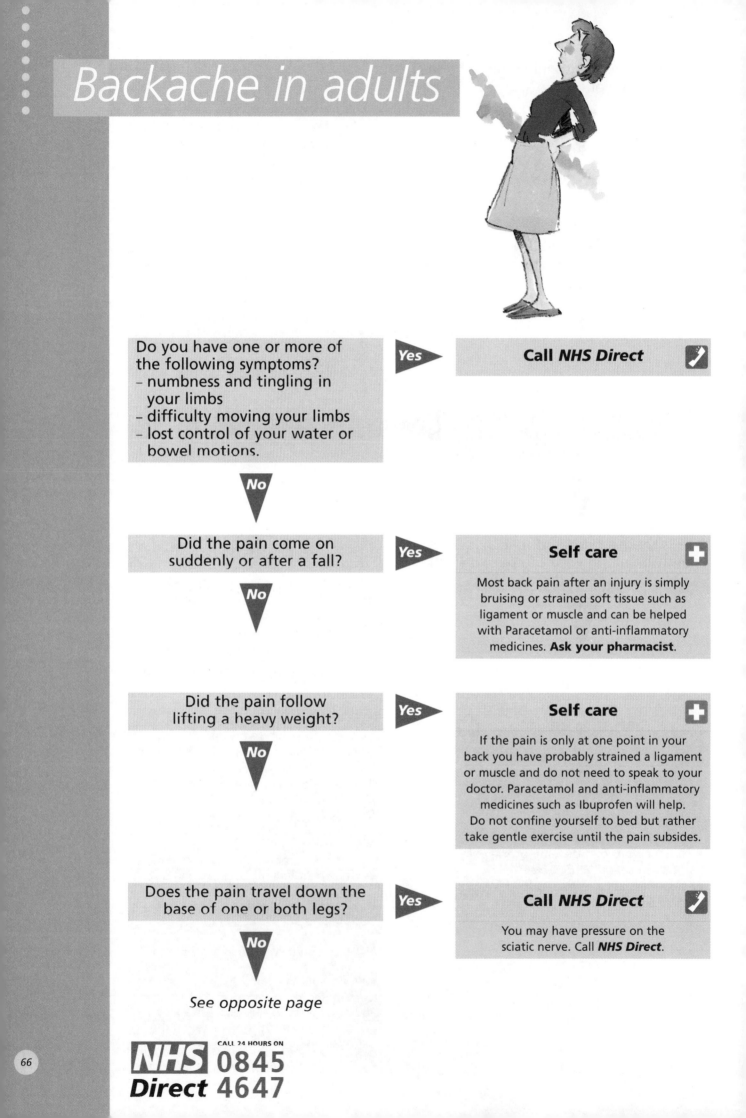

Do you have one or more of the following symptoms?
- numbness and tingling in your limbs
- difficulty moving your limbs
- lost control of your water or bowel motions.

Yes → **Call NHS Direct**

No

Did the pain come on suddenly or after a fall?

Yes → **Self care**

Most back pain after an injury is simply bruising or strained soft tissue such as ligament or muscle and can be helped with Paracetamol or anti-inflammatory medicines. **Ask your pharmacist**.

No

Did the pain follow lifting a heavy weight?

Yes → **Self care**

If the pain is only at one point in your back you have probably strained a ligament or muscle and do not need to speak to your doctor. Paracetamol and anti-inflammatory medicines such as Ibuprofen will help. Do not confine yourself to bed but rather take gentle exercise until the pain subsides.

No

Does the pain travel down the base of one or both legs?

Yes → **Call NHS Direct**

You may have pressure on the sciatic nerve. Call **NHS Direct**.

No

See opposite page

NHS Direct CALL 24 HOURS ON **0845 4647**

Is there also a fever, are you feeling flushed, hot and sweaty (your temperature is over 38°C/100.4°F)?

Yes ▶ **Call *NHS Direct***

No ▼

Does the pain move from the middle of your back to the groin?

Yes ▶ **Call *NHS Direct***

No ▼

Is the pain worse after sitting for prolonged periods?

Yes ▶ **Self care**

Your posture may be wrong and simple painkillers will help. **Ask your pharmacist** for advice.

No ▼

Is the pain tearing or ripping?

Yes ▶ **Call *NHS Direct***

No ▼

Self care advice

- Do not do any lifting but gentle stretching exercises may help.
- Try simple painkillers like Paracetamol or your usual pain relief.
- Avoid medication containing codeine as it may cause constipation.
- Try applying heat packs or ice packs to the area, for no longer than 30 minutes at a time. Repeat every couple of hours. Ice packs should be wrapped in a tea towel to avoid contact with the skin.
- If the condition gets worse or new symptoms develop, call ***NHS Direct***.
- If you are still worried, call ***NHS Direct***.

We'll take the worry away

Chest pain in adults

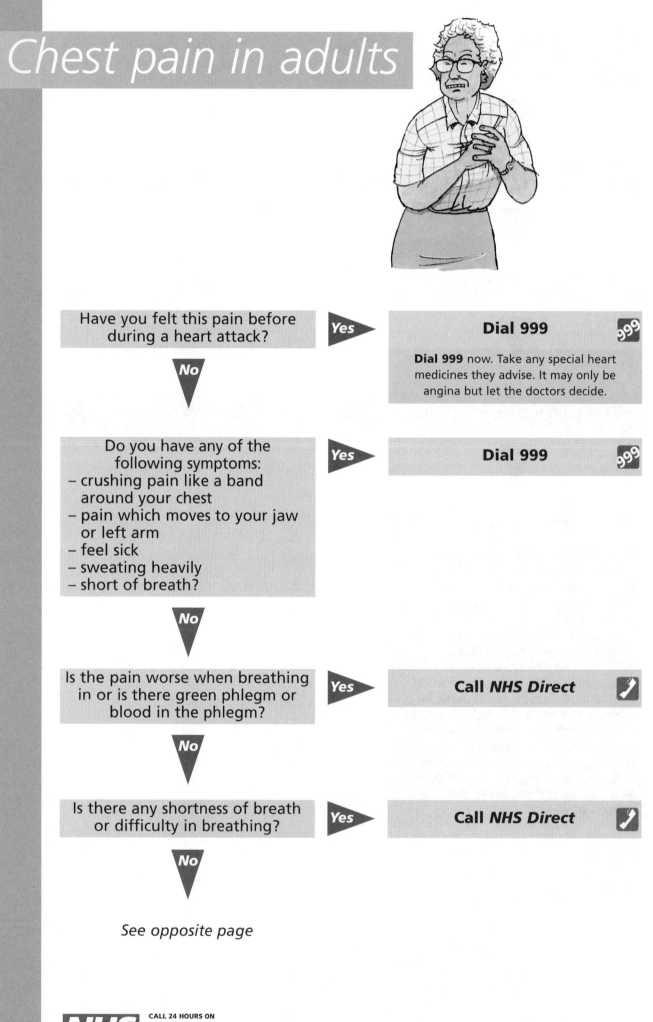

Have you felt this pain before during a heart attack?

Yes → **Dial 999**

Dial 999 now. Take any special heart medicines they advise. It may only be angina but let the doctors decide.

No ↓

Do you have any of the following symptoms:
– crushing pain like a band around your chest
– pain which moves to your jaw or left arm
– feel sick
– sweating heavily
– short of breath?

Yes → **Dial 999**

No ↓

Is the pain worse when breathing in or is there green phlegm or blood in the phlegm?

Yes → **Call NHS Direct**

No ↓

Is there any shortness of breath or difficulty in breathing?

Yes → **Call NHS Direct**

No ↓

See opposite page

NHS Direct
CALL 24 HOURS ON
0845 4647

Is the pain relieved by
indigestion remedies (antacids)?

 Yes

Self care

It may be indigestion. Take any indigestion
remedies or ask your pharmacist who will
give good advice. If the pain fails to settle
within 15 minutes, call **NHS Direct**.

 No

Is the pain worse
when you bend over?

Yes

Call **NHS Direct**

Go to **Hiatus hernia** page 107
for more information

 No

Is the pain worse when you
move your arms or have you
done any unusual or strenuous
exercise recently?

Yes

Self care

You probably have muscle strain.
Ask your pharmacist for advice.

No

If you cannot sort out
what to do from this list,
please, call **NHS Direct**.

NHS CALL 24 HOURS ON
Direct 0845
4647

We'll take the worry away

Diarrhoea in babies and children

*Before going through the following questions check
'How do I know when my baby is ill?'
on page 6*

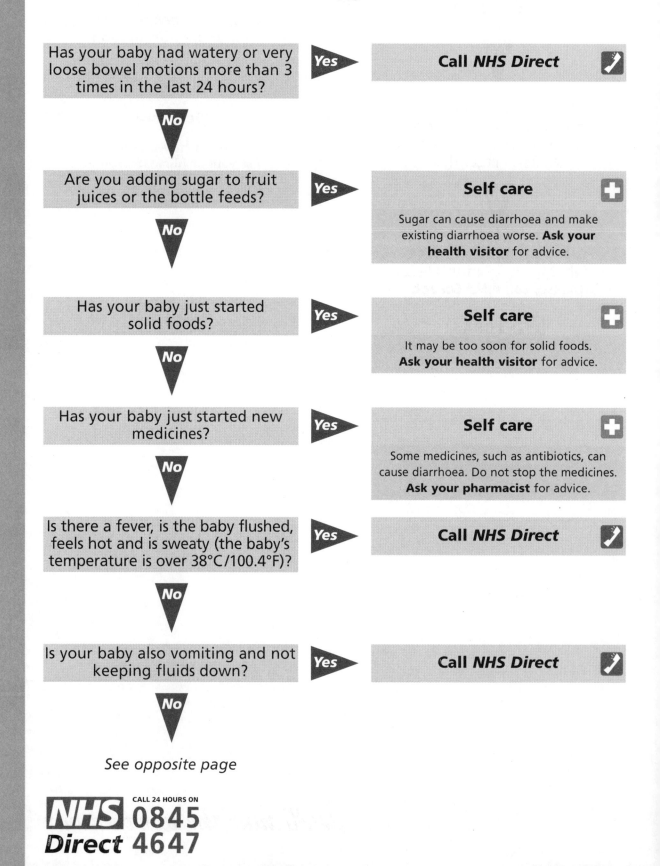

Has your baby had watery or very loose bowel motions more than 3 times in the last 24 hours?

Yes → **Call NHS Direct**

No

Are you adding sugar to fruit juices or the bottle feeds?

Yes → **Self care**

Sugar can cause diarrhoea and make existing diarrhoea worse. **Ask your health visitor** for advice.

No

Has your baby just started solid foods?

Yes → **Self care**

It may be too soon for solid foods. **Ask your health visitor** for advice.

No

Has your baby just started new medicines?

Yes → **Self care**

Some medicines, such as antibiotics, can cause diarrhoea. Do not stop the medicines. **Ask your pharmacist** for advice.

No

Is there a fever, is the baby flushed, feels hot and is sweaty (the baby's temperature is over 38°C/100.4°F)?

Yes → **Call NHS Direct**

No

Is your baby also vomiting and not keeping fluids down?

Yes → **Call NHS Direct**

No

See opposite page

NHS Direct
CALL 24 HOURS ON
0845 4647

| Is there blood in the diarrhoea? | **Yes** | **Call *NHS Direct*** |

No

Self care advice

- Watery or very loose bowel motions are common in babies and young children. If the baby is otherwise well it is likely that the diarrhoea will settle within 24 hours.
- It depends how thirsty the baby/child is as to how much fluid they need.
- *For breast fed babies:*
  - Continue to feed on demand
  - Extra drinks or rehydration fluids (e.g. Dioralyte) from your pharmacist can also be given between feeds
  - For more detailed advice ask your health visitor.
- *For bottle fed babies:*
  - Offer as much fluids or oral rehydration fluids (e.g. dioralyte) as your baby demands for the first 4 hours
  - If diarrhoea continues alternate between the bottle feed and oral rehydration fluids for the next 8 hours
  - Then introduce normal feeds
  - For more detailed advice ask your health visitor.
- *For older children:*
  - Avoid giving solid foods until the child's appetite has returned
  - Offer as much fluid as the child demands (avoid cow's milk for 24 hours until the diarrhoea settles down)
  - Oral re-hydration fluids (e.g. dioralyte) available from your pharmacist will also help
- If any new symptoms develop or the condition gets worse, call ***NHS Direct***.
- If you are still worried, call ***NHS Direct***.

Before ringing *NHS Direct* or 999, it would be helpful if you think about the following and are ready to answer the questions if asked:
- The symptoms (the questions you answered yes to)
- Their temperature (if possible)
- When they last had anything to drink or eat
- Any medicines they are taking at present
- Any allergies you know of
- Any serious illnesses they have had before.

We'll take the worry away

Diarrhoea in adults

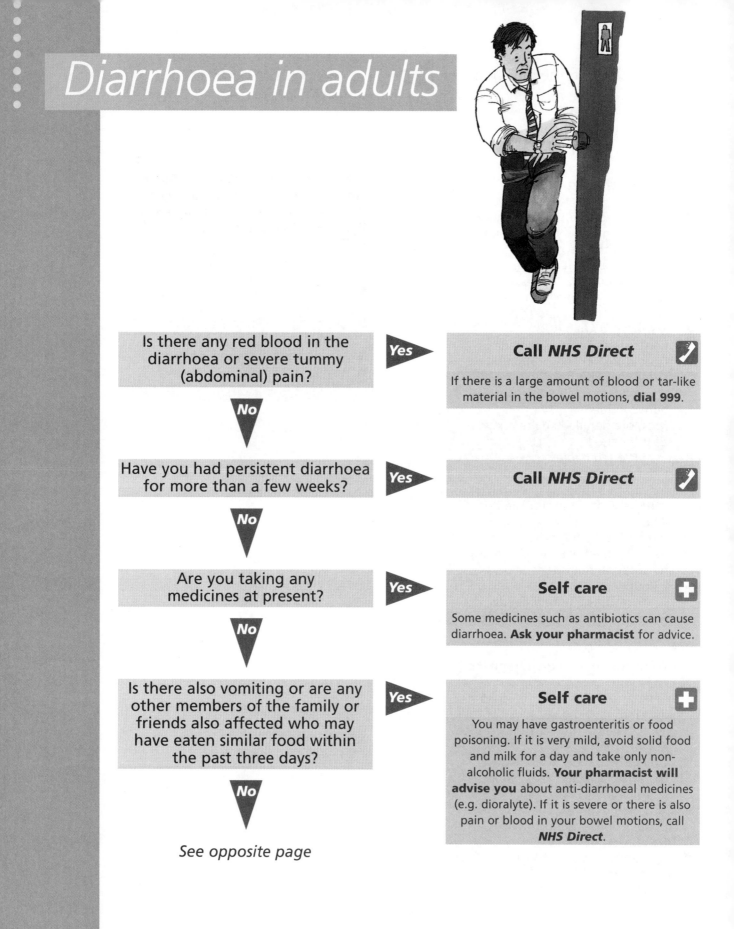

Is there any red blood in the diarrhoea or severe tummy (abdominal) pain?

Yes ➤ **Call NHS Direct**

If there is a large amount of blood or tar-like material in the bowel motions, **dial 999**.

No

Have you had persistent diarrhoea for more than a few weeks?

Yes ➤ **Call NHS Direct**

No

Are you taking any medicines at present?

Yes ➤ **Self care**

Some medicines such as antibiotics can cause diarrhoea. **Ask your pharmacist** for advice.

No

Is there also vomiting or are any other members of the family or friends also affected who may have eaten similar food within the past three days?

Yes ➤ **Self care**

You may have gastroenteritis or food poisoning. If it is very mild, avoid solid food and milk for a day and take only non-alcoholic fluids. **Your pharmacist will advise you** about anti-diarrhoeal medicines (e.g. dioralyte). If it is severe or there is also pain or blood in your bowel motions, call **NHS Direct**.

No

See opposite page

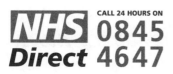

NHS CALL 24 HOURS ON
Direct 0845 4647

Self care advice

- Drink clear fluids only for 24 hours e.g. water.
- Oral rehydration fluids (e.g. dioralyte) are available from your pharmacist and may help.
- Introduce soft, bland foods such as potatoes, bread, dry biscuits in small amounts.
- Once your bowel motions are more solid you can start eating your usual diet.
- Avoid fruit and foods containing roughage such as bran until your diarrhoea has ceased.
- If the condition gets worse or new symptoms develop, call **NHS Direct**.
- If you are still worried, call **NHS Direct**.

Before ringing *NHS Direct* or 999, it would be helpful if you think about the following and are ready to answer the questions if asked:

- The symptoms (the questions you answered yes to)
- If you/they have travelled abroad recently
- Your/their temperature (if possible)
- When you/they last had anything to drink or eat
- Any medicines you/they are taking at present
- Any allergies you know of
- Any serious illnesses you/they have had before.

We'll take the worry away

Female urinary and vaginal problems in adults

For Vaginal bleeding *see page 80*

Are you passing water more often than usual and does it sting each time?

Yes

Self care

You may have a bladder (water) infection (cystitis). Drink plenty of fluids and take Paracetamol. A covered hot water bottle on your tummy also helps. If there is no improvement after two days, call **NHS Direct**.

No

Are you passing blood in your water?

Yes

Call *NHS Direct*

No

Is there a creamy white vaginal discharge or itchiness?

Yes

Self care

You may have thrush (Candida). **See your pharmacist**. If you have repeated attacks over a short space of time, call **NHS Direct**.

Go to *Thrush* page 122 for more information

No

Is there a smelly green/yellow vaginal discharge or itchiness?

Yes

Call *NHS Direct*

No

See opposite page

NHS Direct
CALL 24 HOURS ON
0845 4647

Is there a fever, are you feeling flushed, hot and sweaty (your temperature is over 38°C/100.4°F) or brown blood clots in your urine and a severe pain in your lower back?

Yes → **Call NHS Direct**

No ↓

Are you also experiencing vaginal bleeding?

Yes → Go to *Vaginal bleeding* page 80 for more information ▷

No ↓

Self care advice ✚

- Avoid sexual intercourse until the problem is sorted out.
- Increase your fluid intake to at least 8 glasses of fluid a day. Juices such as Barley water and Cranberry may help.
- Over-the-counter medicines from your pharmacist may also help. They will be able to advise you.
- Avoid use of soap for bathing as this can cause irritation. Take showers if possible.
- Observe the area around the vagina for signs of soreness in which case call **NHS Direct**.
- If new symptoms develop or if your condition worsens, call **NHS Direct**.
- If you are still worried, call **NHS Direct**.

Before ringing **NHS Direct** or **999**, it would be helpful if you think about the following and are ready to answer the questions if asked:
- How long you/they have been unwell
- Your/their temperature (if possible)
- If there is severe back pain which moves to the groin
- Any medicines you/they are taking at present.

Female urinary and vaginal problems in adults

We'll take the worry away

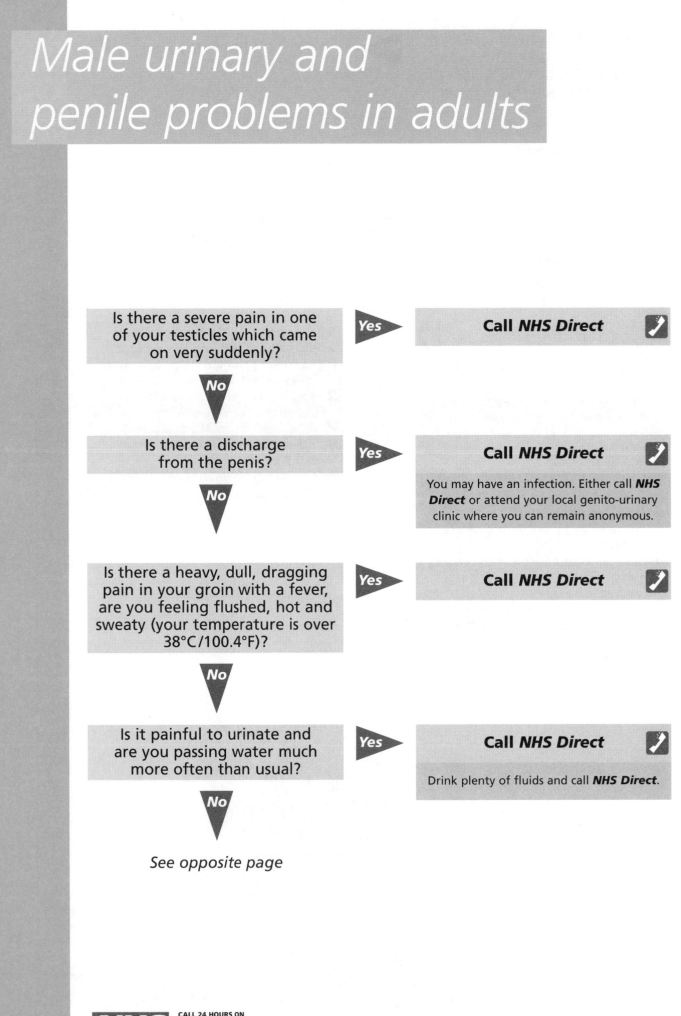

Is there a severe pain in one of your testicles which came on very suddenly?

Yes → **Call NHS Direct**

No ↓

Is there a discharge from the penis?

Yes → **Call NHS Direct**

You may have an infection. Either call **NHS Direct** or attend your local genito-urinary clinic where you can remain anonymous.

No ↓

Is there a heavy, dull, dragging pain in your groin with a fever, are you feeling flushed, hot and sweaty (your temperature is over 38°C/100.4°F)?

Yes → **Call NHS Direct**

No ↓

Is it painful to urinate and are you passing water much more often than usual?

Yes → **Call NHS Direct**

Drink plenty of fluids and call **NHS Direct**.

No ↓

See opposite page

NHS Direct CALL 24 HOURS ON **0845 4647**

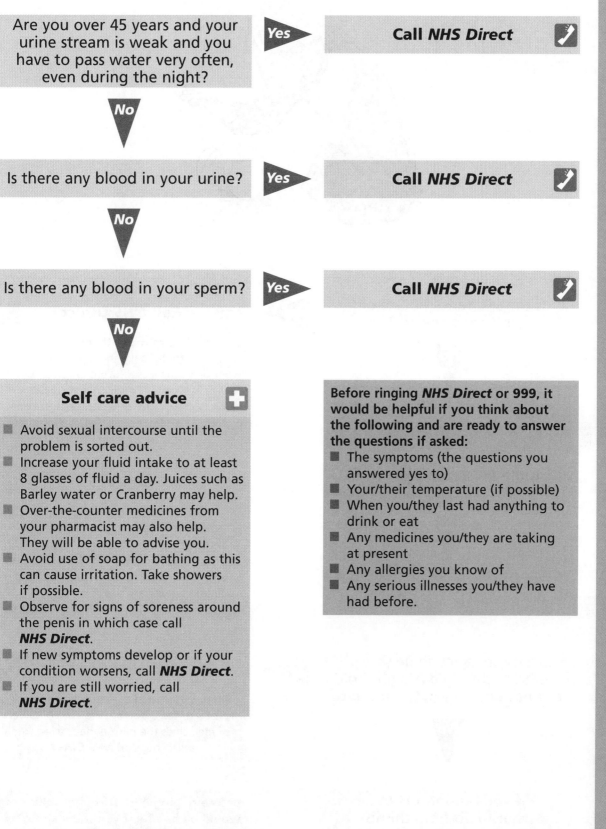

Are you over 45 years and your urine stream is weak and you have to pass water very often, even during the night?

Yes → **Call NHS Direct**

No

Is there any blood in your urine?

Yes → **Call NHS Direct**

No

Is there any blood in your sperm?

Yes → **Call NHS Direct**

No

Self care advice

- Avoid sexual intercourse until the problem is sorted out.
- Increase your fluid intake to at least 8 glasses of fluid a day. Juices such as Barley water or Cranberry may help.
- Over-the-counter medicines from your pharmacist may also help. They will be able to advise you.
- Avoid use of soap for bathing as this can cause irritation. Take showers if possible.
- Observe for signs of soreness around the penis in which case call **NHS Direct**.
- If new symptoms develop or if your condition worsens, call **NHS Direct**.
- If you are still worried, call **NHS Direct**.

Before ringing NHS Direct or 999, it would be helpful if you think about the following and are ready to answer the questions if asked:
- The symptoms (the questions you answered yes to)
- Your/their temperature (if possible)
- When you/they last had anything to drink or eat
- Any medicines you/they are taking at present
- Any allergies you know of
- Any serious illnesses you/they have had before.

We'll take the worry away

Poisoning

This advice is suitable for adults and children

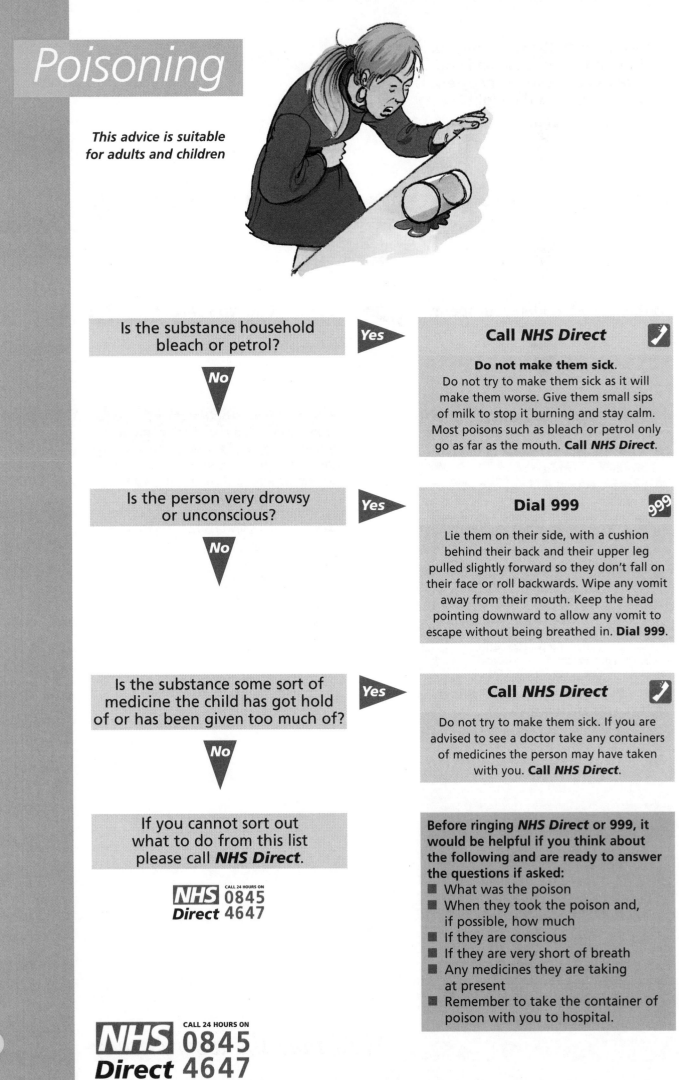

Is the substance household bleach or petrol?

Yes → **Call *NHS Direct***

Do not make them sick.
Do not try to make them sick as it will make them worse. Give them small sips of milk to stop it burning and stay calm. Most poisons such as bleach or petrol only go as far as the mouth. **Call *NHS Direct*.**

No ↓

Is the person very drowsy or unconscious?

Yes → **Dial 999** 999

Lie them on their side, with a cushion behind their back and their upper leg pulled slightly forward so they don't fall on their face or roll backwards. Wipe any vomit away from their mouth. Keep the head pointing downward to allow any vomit to escape without being breathed in. **Dial 999.**

No ↓

Is the substance some sort of medicine the child has got hold of or has been given too much of?

Yes → **Call *NHS Direct***

Do not try to make them sick. If you are advised to see a doctor take any containers of medicines the person may have taken with you. **Call *NHS Direct*.**

No ↓

If you cannot sort out what to do from this list please call *NHS Direct*.

NHS Direct CALL 24 HOURS ON **0845 4647**

Before ringing *NHS Direct* or 999, it would be helpful if you think about the following and are ready to answer the questions if asked:
- What was the poison
- When they took the poison and, if possible, how much
- If they are conscious
- If they are very short of breath
- Any medicines they are taking at present
- Remember to take the container of poison with you to hospital.

NHS Direct CALL 24 HOURS ON **0845 4647**

Self care advice

- Lock all chemicals and medicines away in a child-proof container.

- Keep all products in their original containers. Never put any medicines or chemicals such as weed-killer in soft drink bottles.

- Never refer to medicines as sweets.

- Clean out old medicines frequently and return them for safe destruction to your local community pharmacist.

- Rinse empty containers and throw them out in a safe place.

- Never take or give any medicines in the dark.

- Wherever possible buy products that have child resistant caps.

- Store cleaning products out of reach and where possible out of sight of children.

- Don't store medicines or cleaning agents near food.

- Keep the number of the local poisons unit, your family doctor and your local hospital ready to hand.

- Try taking a safety tour of your home with any young children and see if you can get them to point out the poisons.

- Ask the Royal Society for the Prevention of Accidents for advice on 0121 248 2000.

Below is a list of products that could be dangerous:

- Dish washing liquid
- Scouring soap
- Window cleaner
- Oven cleaner
- Medicines
- Vitamins
- Furniture polish
- Drain cleaner
- Ammonia
- Washing powder
- Bleach
- Fabric softener
- Dye

- Rat/ant poisons
- Moth balls

- Petrol
- Car wax/soaps
- Weedkiller/pesticides
- Paint
- Windscreen washer fluid
- Antifreeze

- Cosmetic products
- Shampoo
- Medications
- Cleansers
- Perfume
- Medicines/painkillers

We'll take the worry away

Adult vaginal bleeding

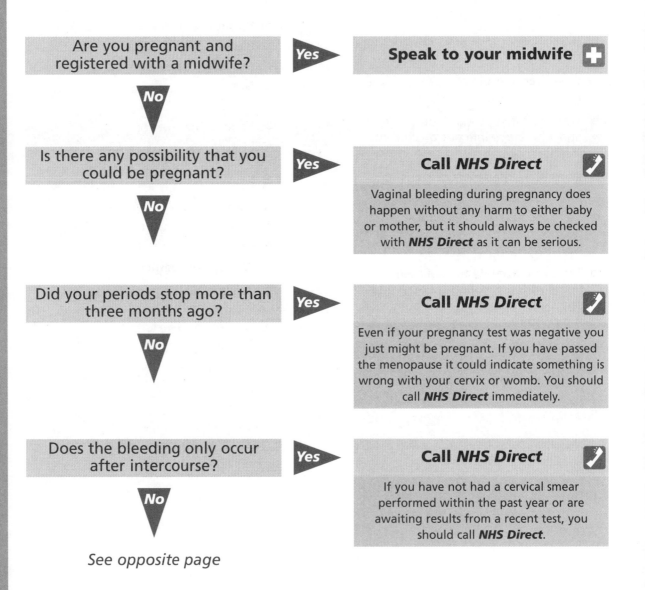

Are you pregnant and registered with a midwife?

Yes → **Speak to your midwife** ✚

No ↓

Is there any possibility that you could be pregnant?

Yes → **Call *NHS Direct*** ✎

Vaginal bleeding during pregnancy does happen without any harm to either baby or mother, but it should always be checked with ***NHS Direct*** as it can be serious.

No ↓

Did your periods stop more than three months ago?

Yes → **Call *NHS Direct*** ✎

Even if your pregnancy test was negative you just might be pregnant. If you have passed the menopause it could indicate something is wrong with your cervix or womb. You should call ***NHS Direct*** immediately.

No ↓

Does the bleeding only occur after intercourse?

Yes → **Call *NHS Direct*** ✎

If you have not had a cervical smear performed within the past year or are awaiting results from a recent test, you should call ***NHS Direct***.

No ↓

See opposite page

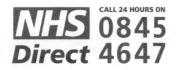

NHS Direct
CALL 24 HOURS ON
0845 4647

Are you taking an oral contraceptive and have changed the type recently?

Yes

Call *NHS Direct*

Breakthrough bleeding is common especially when the oral contraceptive pill has recently been changed, if you have been ill, are vomiting or have diarrhoea. If it continues, see your family planning advisor or your doctor. Call *NHS Direct*.

No

Have you only just started having periods within the past three years?

Yes

Call *NHS Direct*

Irregular periods are very common as you approach puberty (the start of periods). If they continue to be irregular, call *NHS Direct*.

No

Did you think you had started or are approaching the change of life (menopause)?

Yes

Call *NHS Direct*

Periods often become irregular as you approach the change of life (menopause) but there should never be any bleeding after you have been through the menopause. If there is bleeding, call *NHS Direct*.

No

Is there severe pain or do you have an intrauterine contraceptive device (coil) or are you 3 months pregnant?

Yes

Call *NHS Direct*

There is a possibility of a pregnancy outside the normal place within the womb. This is a greater possibility if you have ever had a serious infection of the womb or if you have had a sterilisation reversed. Call *NHS Direct*.

No

Self care advice ✚

- Try resting and keep a record of the towels/tampons you use. This will help to assess the amount of blood loss.
- Take painkillers such as Paracetamol if you have pain or discomfort.
- You will need to book a routine appointment with your GP if this is happening regularly.
- If any new symptoms develop or the conditions worsens, call *NHS Direct*.
- If you are still worried, call *NHS Direct*.

Before ringing *NHS Direct* or 999, it would be helpful if you think about the following and are ready to answer the questions if asked:
- Where the pain is
- Any previous pregnancies
- Date of your/their last period
- Information on the contraception you/they use
- If you/they have had a pregnancy test – when and what was the result
- Results of your last cervical smear
- Your/their temperature (if possible).

We'll take the worry away

Vomiting in babies

Before going through the following questions check 'How do I know when my baby is ill?' on page 6

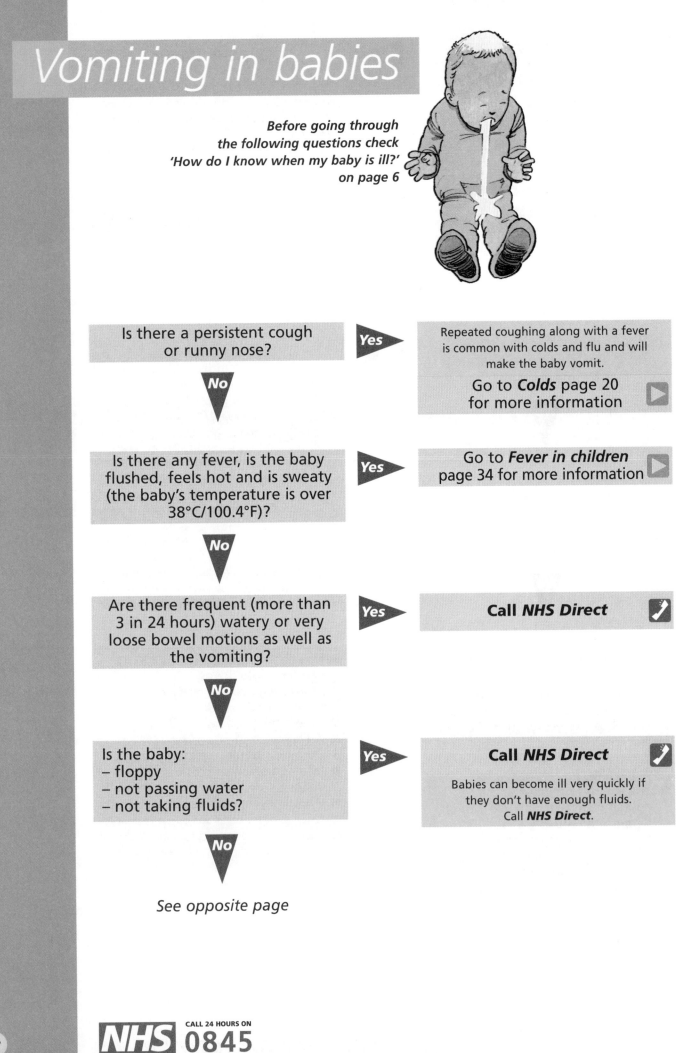

Is there a persistent cough or runny nose? → **Yes** → Repeated coughing along with a fever is common with colds and flu and will make the baby vomit.

Go to *Colds* page 20 for more information ▶

No ▼

Is there any fever, is the baby flushed, feels hot and is sweaty (the baby's temperature is over 38°C/100.4°F)? → **Yes** → **Go to *Fever in children* page 34 for more information** ▶

No ▼

Are there frequent (more than 3 in 24 hours) watery or very loose bowel motions as well as the vomiting? → **Yes** → **Call *NHS Direct***

No ▼

Is the baby:
– floppy
– not passing water
– not taking fluids? → **Yes** → **Call *NHS Direct***

Babies can become ill very quickly if they don't have enough fluids. Call ***NHS Direct***.

No ▼

See opposite page

NHS Direct

CALL 24 HOURS ON
0845 4647

Is the vomiting forceful (projectile) and after each feed or is there weight loss?

Yes

Call *NHS Direct*

There may be a problem with the emptying of the stomach. Call **NHS Direct**.

No

Is the vomiting just small amounts after feeds and the baby is otherwise fine?

Yes

Self care

Babies often bring up small amounts of their feed but it should look similar to their milk feed and not come out with any force. Winding helps. Using an over large hole in the teat when bottle feeding is a common cause. Avoid over use of 'colic treatments'.

No

Is the baby crying continuously or obviously in pain?

Yes

Call *NHS Direct*

It can be difficult to tell when a baby is in severe pain as well as vomiting. A change in the way the baby is crying, particularly when previously well, or if there is a rash or fever, call **NHS Direct**.

No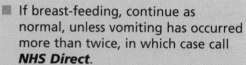

Self care advice

- If breast-feeding, continue as normal, unless vomiting has occurred more than twice, in which case call **NHS Direct**.
- If bottle-feeding, introduce rehydration fluids (e.g. Dioralyte) in small quantities as per the manufacturer's instructions on the package. Speak to your pharmacist.
- Do not give large amounts of fluids in one go and reintroduce milk gradually.
- If the condition has not improved within 2 hours or the baby does not have a wet nappy or other symptoms have developed, call **NHS Direct**.
- If you are still worried, call **NHS Direct**.

Before ringing *NHS Direct* or 999, it would be helpful if you think about the following and are ready to answer the questions if asked:
- The symptoms (the questions you answered yes to)
- Their temperature (if possible)
- When they last had anything to drink or eat
- Any medicines they are taking at present
- Any allergies you know of
- Any serious illnesses they have had before.

Vomiting in babies

We'll take the worry away

Vomiting in children

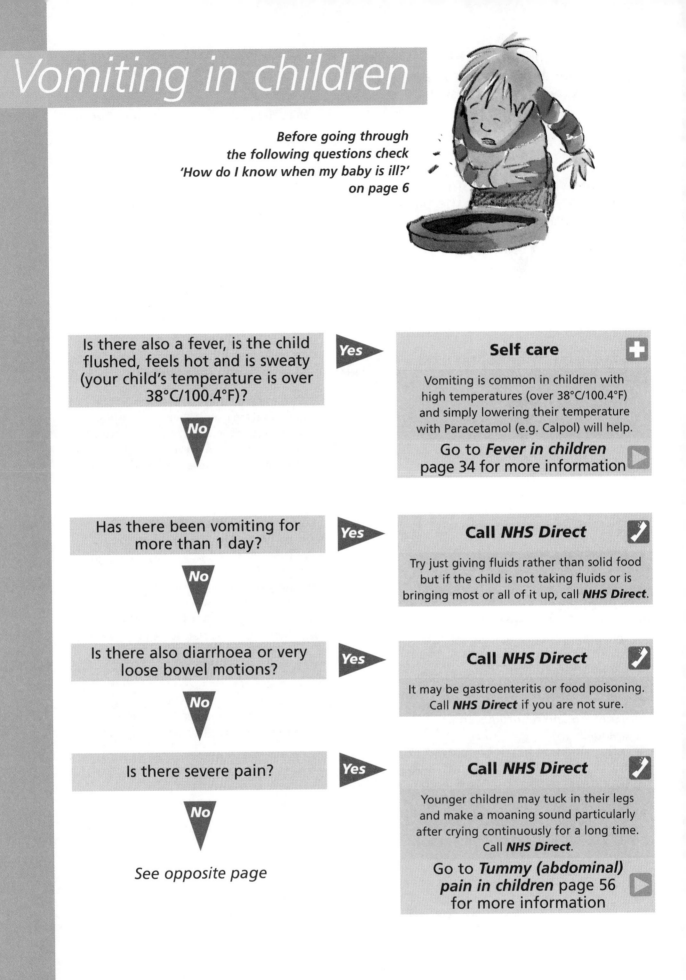

*Before going through
the following questions check
'How do I know when my baby is ill?'
on page 6*

Is there also a fever, is the child flushed, feels hot and is sweaty (your child's temperature is over 38°C/100.4°F)?

Yes →

Self care

Vomiting is common in children with high temperatures (over 38°C/100.4°F) and simply lowering their temperature with Paracetamol (e.g. Calpol) will help.

Go to *Fever in children* page 34 for more information

No ↓

Has there been vomiting for more than 1 day?

Yes →

Call *NHS Direct*

Try just giving fluids rather than solid food but if the child is not taking fluids or is bringing most or all of it up, call *NHS Direct*.

No ↓

Is there also diarrhoea or very loose bowel motions?

Yes →

Call *NHS Direct*

It may be gastroenteritis or food poisoning. Call *NHS Direct* if you are not sure.

No ↓

Is there severe pain?

Yes →

Call *NHS Direct*

Younger children may tuck in their legs and make a moaning sound particularly after crying continuously for a long time. Call *NHS Direct*.

Go to *Tummy (abdominal) pain in children* page 56 for more information

No ↓

See opposite page

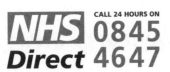

NHS Direct CALL 24 HOURS ON **0845 4647**

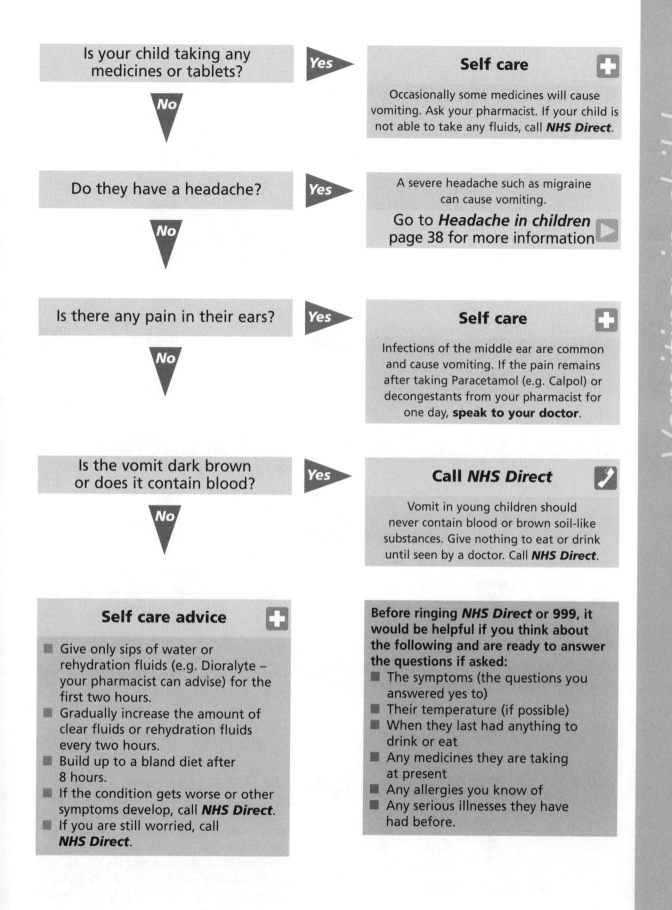

Is your child taking any medicines or tablets?

Yes

No

Self care

Occasionally some medicines will cause vomiting. Ask your pharmacist. If your child is not able to take any fluids, call **NHS Direct**.

Do they have a headache?

Yes

No

A severe headache such as migraine can cause vomiting.

Go to Headache in children page 38 for more information

Is there any pain in their ears?

Yes

No

Self care

Infections of the middle ear are common and cause vomiting. If the pain remains after taking Paracetamol (e.g. Calpol) or decongestants from your pharmacist for one day, **speak to your doctor**.

Is the vomit dark brown or does it contain blood?

Yes

No

Call NHS Direct

Vomit in young children should never contain blood or brown soil-like substances. Give nothing to eat or drink until seen by a doctor. Call **NHS Direct**.

Self care advice

- Give only sips of water or rehydration fluids (e.g. Dioralyte – your pharmacist can advise) for the first two hours.
- Gradually increase the amount of clear fluids or rehydration fluids every two hours.
- Build up to a bland diet after 8 hours.
- If the condition gets worse or other symptoms develop, call **NHS Direct**.
- If you are still worried, call **NHS Direct**.

Before ringing **NHS Direct** or 999, it would be helpful if you think about the following and are ready to answer the questions if asked:
- The symptoms (the questions you answered yes to)
- Their temperature (if possible)
- When they last had anything to drink or eat
- Any medicines they are taking at present
- Any allergies you know of
- Any serious illnesses they have had before.

We'll take the worry away

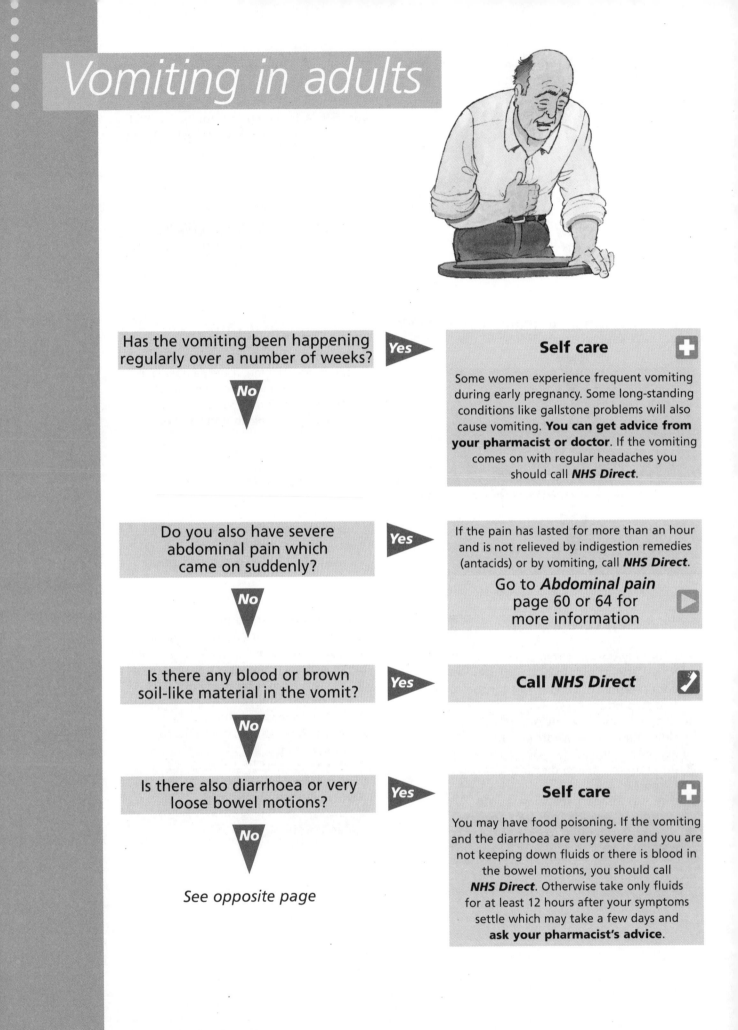

Has the vomiting been happening regularly over a number of weeks?

Yes

No

Self care

Some women experience frequent vomiting during early pregnancy. Some long-standing conditions like gallstone problems will also cause vomiting. **You can get advice from your pharmacist or doctor**. If the vomiting comes on with regular headaches you should call **NHS Direct**.

Do you also have severe abdominal pain which came on suddenly?

Yes

No

If the pain has lasted for more than an hour and is not relieved by indigestion remedies (antacids) or by vomiting, call **NHS Direct**.

Go to **Abdominal pain** page 60 or 64 for more information

Is there any blood or brown soil-like material in the vomit?

Yes

No

Call NHS Direct

Is there also diarrhoea or very loose bowel motions?

Yes

No

Self care

You may have food poisoning. If the vomiting and the diarrhoea are very severe and you are not keeping down fluids or there is blood in the bowel motions, you should call **NHS Direct**. Otherwise take only fluids for at least 12 hours after your symptoms settle which may take a few days and **ask your pharmacist's advice**.

See opposite page

NHS Direct
CALL 24 HOURS ON
0845 4647

Do you have a severe headache? **Yes**

No

Dial 999

Any severe pain will cause vomiting but if you do not normally suffer from headaches such as migraine, or there has been a recent head injury, or the light is hurting your eyes, you should **dial 999**.

Self care advice ✚

- Try small amounts of clear fluids or rehydration fluids (e.g. Dioralyte) from your pharmacist.
- Build up the amount of fluids from sips to a cup full over the next 12 hours.
- 12 hours after the last bout of vomiting, introduce bland foods back into your diet (this includes dry biscuits, toast or crackers).
- Avoid milk in your diet during this period.
- Sometimes the cause of vomiting can be bacterial infection, and can be spread to other people.
- It is therefore important to thoroughly clean all areas that have been in contact with the vomit.
- Be extra careful about personal hygiene, washing hands, etc.
- If the condition worsens or new symptoms develop, call **NHS Direct**.
- If you are still worried, call **NHS Direct**.

Before ringing **NHS Direct** or **999**, it would be helpful if you think about the following and are ready to answer the questions if asked:
- The symptoms (the questions you answered yes to)
- Your/their temperature (if possible)
- When you/they last had anything to drink or eat
- Any medicines you/they are taking at present
- Any allergies you know of
- Any serious illnesses you/they have had before.

We'll take the worry away

Injuries to hands and feet

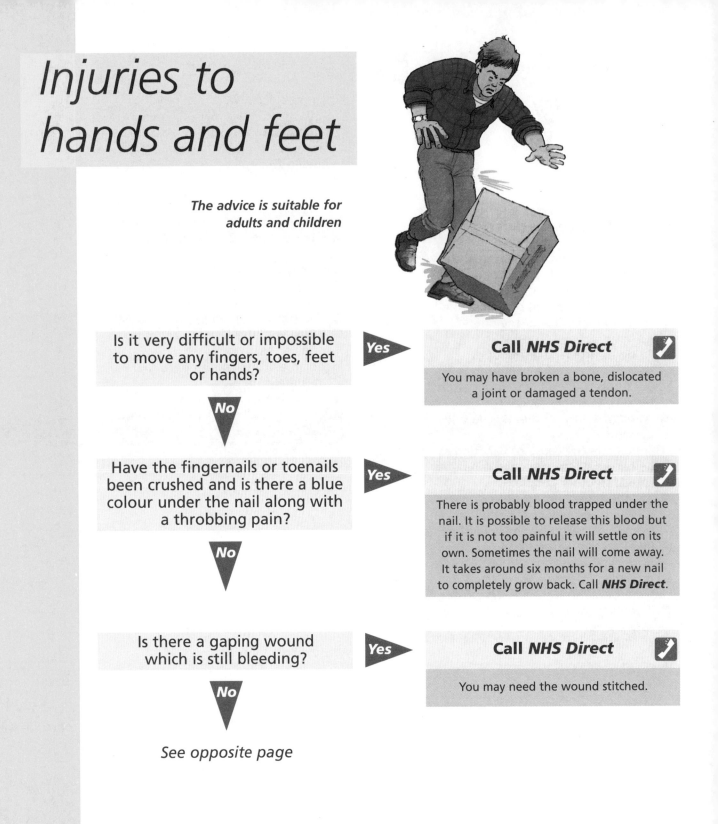

The advice is suitable for adults and children

Is it very difficult or impossible to move any fingers, toes, feet or hands?

Yes → **Call NHS Direct**

You may have broken a bone, dislocated a joint or damaged a tendon.

No ↓

Have the fingernails or toenails been crushed and is there a blue colour under the nail along with a throbbing pain?

Yes → **Call NHS Direct**

There is probably blood trapped under the nail. It is possible to release this blood but if it is not too painful it will settle on its own. Sometimes the nail will come away. It takes around six months for a new nail to completely grow back. Call **NHS Direct**.

No ↓

Is there a gaping wound which is still bleeding?

Yes → **Call NHS Direct**

You may need the wound stitched.

No ↓

See opposite page

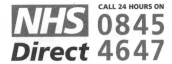

NHS Direct
CALL 24 HOURS ON
0845 4647

Is the cut minor and is it easy to stop the blood from flowing?

 Yes

No

Self care

Clean the wound with tap water and cover with an adhesive plaster or dry bandage. If the person is not covered for tetanus they should contact their GP's surgery.

What to do if you lose a limb or finger or toe?

Dial 999

- Press on the wound with a clean cloth or bandage to stop blood loss.
- Lift the hand or foot higher than waist height.
- If possible lie the person down and lift the foot or hand higher than their chest.
- Put the finger or toe into a plastic bag.
- Put this bag into another bag containing ice.
- Do not let the ice come into direct contact with the finger or toe.
- Take this with you to your local hospital's accident and emergency department and tell the ambulance crew what you have done. It may be possible to sew it back on.

Before ringing *NHS Direct* or 999, it would be helpful if you think about the following and are ready to answer the questions if asked:
- If there is a serious wound with loss of blood
- If there is a serious crush injury and you/they cannot move their fingers or toes
- If any fingers or toes have been completely torn off
- If any bones are sticking out of the wound.

We'll take the worry away

Joint pains

*This advice is suitable for adults. Joint pain in children is uncommon but when it occurs, you should seek advice from **NHS Direct**.*

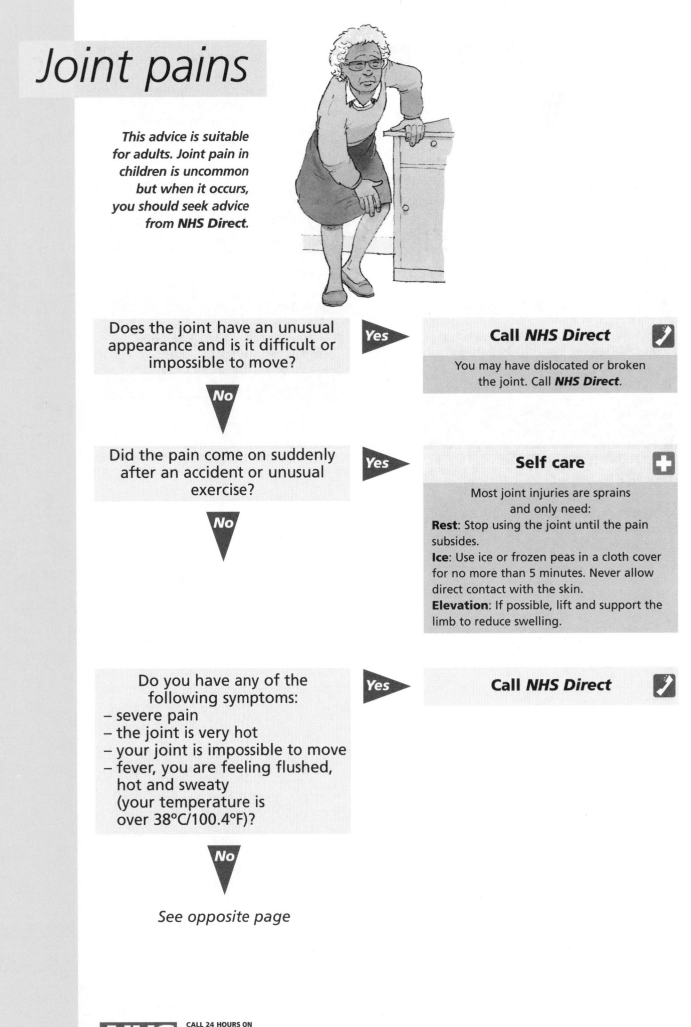

Does the joint have an unusual appearance and is it difficult or impossible to move?

Yes →

Call *NHS Direct*

You may have dislocated or broken the joint. Call **NHS Direct**.

No ↓

Did the pain come on suddenly after an accident or unusual exercise?

Yes →

Self care

Most joint injuries are sprains and only need:

Rest: Stop using the joint until the pain subsides.

Ice: Use ice or frozen peas in a cloth cover for no more than 5 minutes. Never allow direct contact with the skin.

Elevation: If possible, lift and support the limb to reduce swelling.

No ↓

Do you have any of the following symptoms:
– severe pain
– the joint is very hot
– your joint is impossible to move
– fever, you are feeling flushed, hot and sweaty
(your temperature is over 38°C/100.4°F)?

Yes →

Call *NHS Direct*

No ↓

See opposite page

NHS Direct
CALL 24 HOURS ON
0845 4647

Is this the first time you have felt such pain in your joints?

Yes ▶ **Call *NHS Direct***

No ▼

Are other joints hot, swollen and painful as well?

Yes ▶ **Call *NHS Direct***

No ▼

Does the pain follow the same repeated movements like typing, using a screwdriver or playing tennis?

Yes ▶ **Self care** ✚

You may have a repetitive strain injury which will respond to rest or alternative forms of exercise. Anti-inflammatory medicines do help. **Ask your pharmacist** for advice.

No ▼

Does the pain gradually get worse as the day goes on?

Yes ▶ **Self care** ✚

You may have osteoarthritis which is caused by wear and tear. **Ask your pharmacist** for advice.

No ▼

Self care advice ✚

- It is important to rest the affected area.
- Complete rest may make the condition worse.
- Regular painkillers such as Paracetamol or Ibuprofen may help.
- A cold compress will help reduce swelling.
- An ice-pack or bag of frozen peas wrapped in a tea towel can be applied to the area for no longer than 30 minutes. Repeat every 2 hours.
- If the pain continues or new symptoms develop, call ***NHS Direct***.
- If you are still worried, call ***NHS Direct***.

Before ringing ***NHS Direct*** or 999, it would be helpful if you think about the following and are ready to answer the questions if asked:
- How long you/they have been unwell
- Your/their temperature (if possible)
- Any medicines you/they are taking at present
- Any illnesses, such as rheumatoid arthritis, you/they have had before.

We'll take the worry away

Burns & scalds

This advice is suitable for adults and children

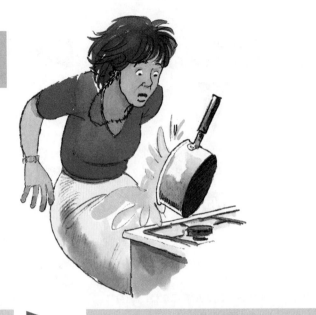

Is there any shortness of breath?	**Yes** ▶	**Dial 999** 999 Inhaling fumes or flame can damage the airways. If they are short of breath, **dial 999**.

No ▼

Are there any other injuries such as electric shock or broken bones?	**Yes** ▶	**Dial 999** 999 If the burn came from an electric shock or there are broken bones from a fall, **dial 999**.

No ▼

Is the burn or scald area larger than the size of the adult's or child's own hand?	**Yes** ▶	**Call *NHS Direct*** It is easy to underestimate the area of a burn or scald. If it is larger than the size of the person's hand, call **NHS Direct**.

No ▼

Is the burn or scald on the face or around the mouth?	**Yes** ▶	**Call *NHS Direct*** Burns or scalds around the mouth may mean that they have inhaled the fumes or flame. Call **NHS Direct**.

No ▼

See opposite page

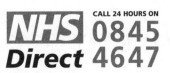 **NHS Direct** CALL 24 HOURS ON **0845 4647**

Do you feel you need further advice on how to treat this burn? **Call *NHS Direct***

No

Self care advice

- Take off any bracelets, rings, shoes, necklaces or watches which may restrict blood flow.
- Cool with running water for 15 minutes.
- Do not apply any creams or ointments.
- Cover with a clean, dry, non-fluffy cotton cloth (for example, a handkerchief).
- Take some painkillers such as Paracetamol.
- If the condition gets worse or new symptoms develop, call ***NHS Direct***.
- If you are still worried, call ***NHS Direct***.

Before ringing *NHS Direct* or 999, it would be helpful if you think about the following and are ready to answer the questions if asked:
- When the burn or scald happened
- If it involved an electric shock
- If they are unconscious
- If there are any broken bones
- The approximate size of the burn or scald.

Burns & scalds

We'll take the worry away

Rashes

This advice is suitable for adults and children

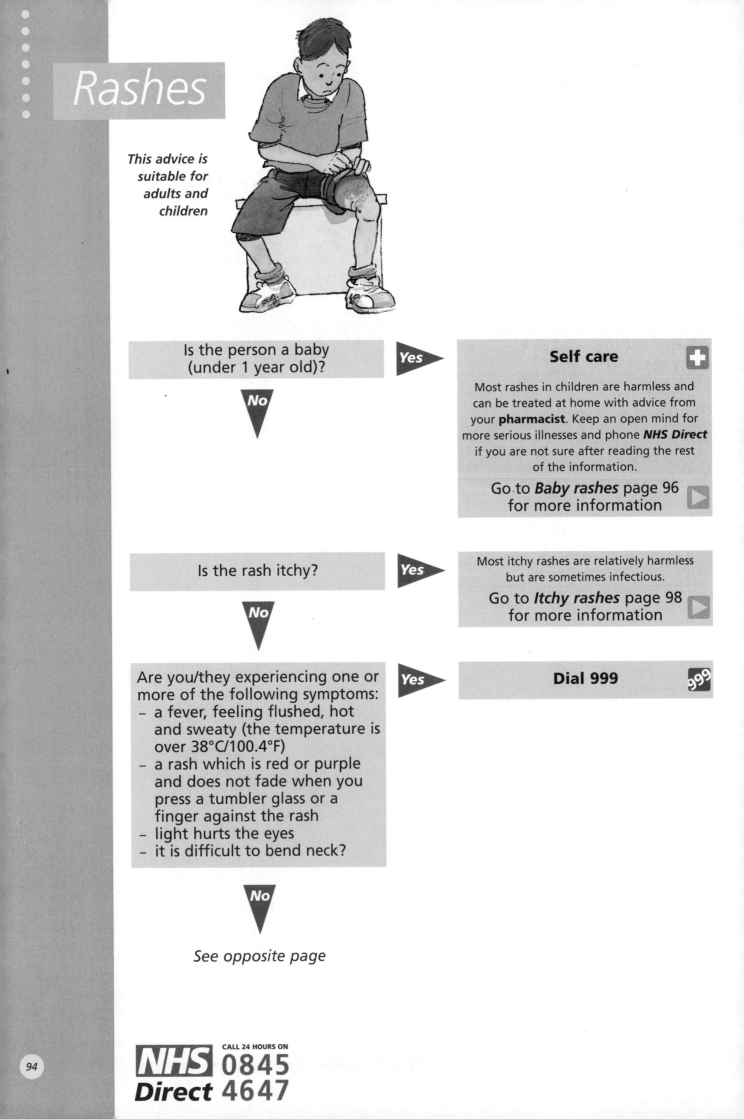

Is the person a baby (under 1 year old)?

Yes ▶

Self care ✚

Most rashes in children are harmless and can be treated at home with advice from your **pharmacist**. Keep an open mind for more serious illnesses and phone **NHS Direct** if you are not sure after reading the rest of the information.

Go to *Baby rashes* page 96 for more information ▶

No ▼

Is the rash itchy?

Yes ▶

Most itchy rashes are relatively harmless but are sometimes infectious.

Go to *Itchy rashes* page 98 for more information ▶

No ▼

Are you/they experiencing one or more of the following symptoms:
- a fever, feeling flushed, hot and sweaty (the temperature is over 38°C/100.4°F)
- a rash which is red or purple and does not fade when you press a tumbler glass or a finger against the rash
- light hurts the eyes
- it is difficult to bend neck?

Yes ▶

Dial 999 999

No ▼

See opposite page

NHS Direct CALL 24 HOURS ON **0845 4647**

Is the rash:
- dark red
- mainly on the elbows, legs, buttocks
- does it come and go?

 Yes ▶

 No

Call *NHS Direct*

Serious problems are rare but these irregularly shaped dark red spots could follow an allergic reaction to infection or some disorder of the blood. Call *NHS Direct*.

Go to *Purpura* page 117 for more information

Is it red and crusty, or are there weeping sores on the face?

Yes ▶

No ▼

Self care ✚

It may be impetigo which is more common in children but is also seen in adults. It is infectious.
Use separate washing materials and ease any pain with Paracetamol (e.g. Calpol for children) (not aspirin in any child under 12 years). If it persists, your doctor can give you a treatment for the infection.

Go to *Impetigo* page 108 for more information ▶

Self care advice ✚

- A rash alone is unlikely to be serious.
- Encourage the person to rest and observe closely for signs of illness.
- Ensure the person is drinking plenty of fluids.
- Paracetamol (e.g. Calpol for children) may be helpful if the person is restless.
- Ask your pharmacist to recommend a cream that may provide some relief.
- Calamine lotion will give relief for a short time.
- 2 tablespoons of sodium bicarbonate (e.g. bicarbonate of soda) added to bath water may relieve any itching.
- If the condition gets worse or if any other symptoms develop, call *NHS Direct*.
- If you are still worried, call *NHS Direct*.

Before ringing *NHS Direct* or 999, it would be helpful if you think about the following and are ready to answer the questions if asked:
- The symptoms (the questions you answered yes to)
- Your/their temperature (if possible)
- When you/they last had anything to drink or eat
- Any medicines you/they are taking at present
- Any allergies you know of
- Any serious illnesses you/they have had before.

We'll take the worry away

Baby rashes

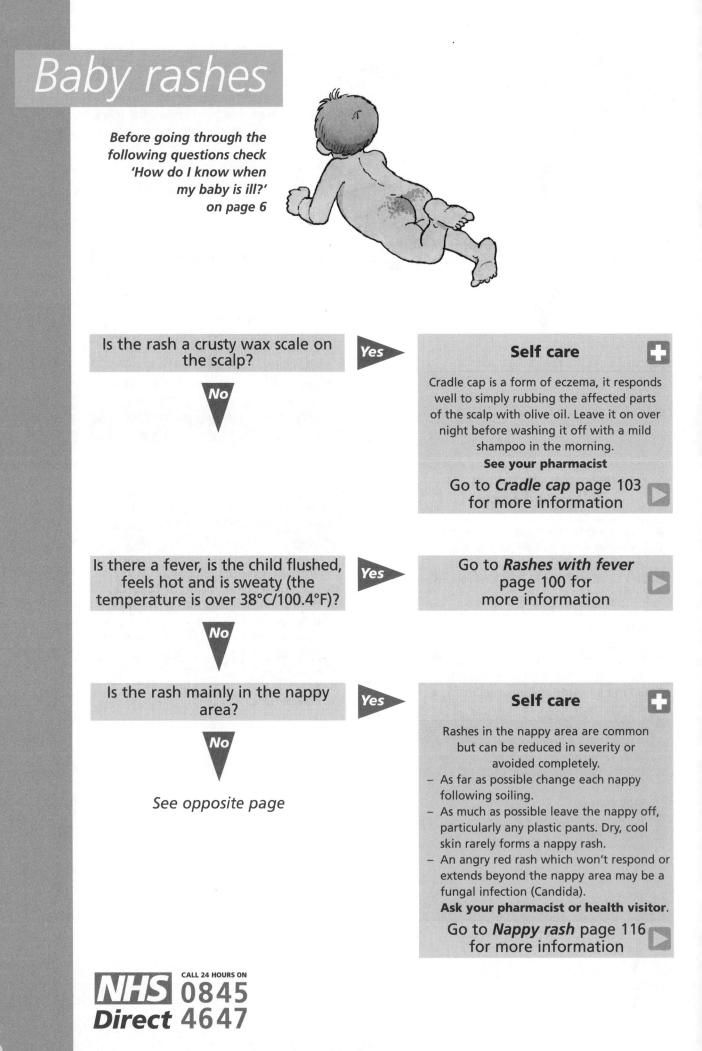

Before going through the following questions check 'How do I know when my baby is ill?' on page 6

Is the rash a crusty wax scale on the scalp?

Yes ▶

Self care ✚

Cradle cap is a form of eczema, it responds well to simply rubbing the affected parts of the scalp with olive oil. Leave it on over night before washing it off with a mild shampoo in the morning.

See your pharmacist

Go to *Cradle cap* page 103 for more information ▶

No ▼

Is there a fever, is the child flushed, feels hot and is sweaty (the temperature is over 38°C/100.4°F)?

Yes ▶

Go to *Rashes with fever* page 100 for more information ▶

No ▼

Is the rash mainly in the nappy area?

Yes ▶

Self care ✚

Rashes in the nappy area are common but can be reduced in severity or avoided completely.

– As far as possible change each nappy following soiling.
– As much as possible leave the nappy off, particularly any plastic pants. Dry, cool skin rarely forms a nappy rash.
– An angry red rash which won't respond or extends beyond the nappy area may be a fungal infection (Candida).

Ask your pharmacist or health visitor.

Go to *Nappy rash* page 116 for more information ▶

No ▼

See opposite page

NHS Direct
CALL 24 HOURS ON
0845 4647

Is the rash red, itchy, flaky and in more than one place? **Yes**

No

Self care

Eczema covers a range of skin problems. There is a wide range of products which will help stop the itchiness and keep the skin moist. Follow your doctor's advice on the use of topical steroid creams.
Call **NHS Direct**, but call your **doctor** if:
– the eczema is spreading very quickly
– the skin is becoming infected
– there is severe pain.

Go to *Eczema* page 104 for more information

Is the rash blotchy, red and difficult to feel? **Yes**

No

Self care

All babies and children will have a heat rash at some time. No treatment is required other than lowering their temperature by moving them from the heat, removing their clothes and keeping them in a cool room.

Go to *Heat rash* page 107 for more information

Is the rash:
– dark red
– mainly on the elbows, legs, buttocks
– does it change its appearance and place on the skin? **Yes**

No

Call *NHS Direct*

Serious problems are rare but these irregularly shaped dark red spots could follow an allergic reaction to infection or some disorder of the blood. Call **NHS Direct**.

Go to *Purpura* page 117 for more information

Self care advice

- A rash alone is unlikely to be serious.
- Encourage the child to rest and observe closely for signs of illness.
- Ensure the child is drinking plenty of fluids.
- Paracetamol (e.g. Calpol) may be helpful if the child is restless.
- Ask your pharmacist to recommend a cream that may provide some relief.
- Calamine lotion will give relief for a short time.
- 2 tablespoons of sodium bicarbonate (e.g. bicarbonate of soda) added to bath water may relieve any itching.
- If the condition gets worse or if any other symptoms develop, call **NHS Direct**.
- If you are still worried, call **NHS Direct**.

Before ringing *NHS Direct* or 999, it would be helpful if you think about the following and are ready to answer the questions if asked:
- The symptoms (the questions you answered yes to)
- Their temperature (if possible)
- When they last had anything to drink or eat.
- Any medicines they are taking at present
- Any allergies you know of
- Any serious illnesses they have had before.

We'll take the worry away

Itchy rashes

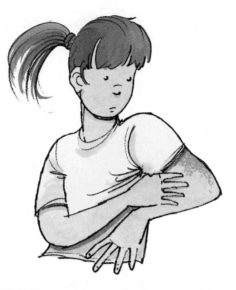

Is the rash red, smooth, slightly raised (you can feel it)?

Yes ▶

No ▼

Self care ✚

Hives can be a reaction to food (e.g. shell fish, strawberries), medicines, plants (e.g. nettles) or a viral infection. The rash will usually disappear in a few hours without any treatment. Call **NHS Direct** if the rash has not disappeared after 24 hours. **Dial 999** if there are any breathing difficulties or they cannot swallow.

Go to *Hives & Urticaria* page 108 for more information ▷

Is the rash only at the lips and mouth corners?

Yes ▶

No ▼

See opposite page

Self care ✚

It could be a cold sore.
- Once infected, avoid sudden changes in temperature and sun exposure.
- Use simple painkillers such as Paracetamol (e.g. Calpol, not aspirin in children under 12 years).
- Use a lip salve before going into bright sunlight.
- Aciclovir cream (e.g. Zovirax) from your **pharmacist** will limit the outbreak.

Go to *Cold sores* page 103 for more information ▷

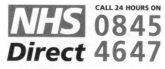

NHS Direct CALL 24 HOURS ON **0845 4647**

Is the rash shaped like a ring and is flaky? **Yes**

No

Self care

Ringworm (Tinea) can affect many parts of the body, particularly the groin and scalp. Keep the area well ventilated and dry. Use an antifungal cream or shampoo available from your **pharmacist** and keep your face cloth and towel separate. Ringworm is infectious.

Go to *Ringworm* page 118 for more information

Is the rash itchy, on the fingers, hand or wrist? **Yes**

No

Self care

Scabies is caused by a mite which burrows just under the skin, often between the fingers, wrists, elbows and the genital areas. Ointments are available from your **pharmacist**. The body from the neck down will need to be covered with the ointment for 24 hours and all clothing and bedding should be washed thoroughly.

Go to *Scabies* page 118 for more information

Is it raised with one or more in the same area? **Yes**

No

Self care

At first insect bites can be mistaken for more serious things. If you look very closely you can generally see the small hole of the actual bite. **See your pharmacist**.

Go to *Insect bites* page 110 for more information

Self care advice

- A rash alone is unlikely to be serious.
- Encourage the child to rest and observe closely for signs of illness.
- Ensure the child is drinking plenty of fluids.
- Paracetamol (e.g. Calpol) may be helpful if the child is restless.
- Ask your pharmacist to recommend a cream that may provide some relief.
- Calamine lotion will give relief for a short time.
- 2 tablespoons of sodium bicarbonate (e.g. bicarbonate of soda) added to bath water may relieve any itching.
- If the condition gets worse or if any other symptoms develop, call **NHS Direct**.
- If you are still worried, call **NHS Direct**.

Before ringing *NHS Direct* or 999, it would be helpful if you think about the following and are ready to answer the questions if asked:
- The symptoms (the questions you answered yes to)
- Your/their temperature (if possible)
- When you/they last had anything to drink or eat.
- Any medicines you/they are taking at present
- Any allergies you know of
- Any serious illnesses you/they have had before.

We'll take the worry away

Rashes with fever

You/they may have a fever, if you/they are feeling flushed, hot and sweaty (your/their temperature is over 38°C/100.4°F)

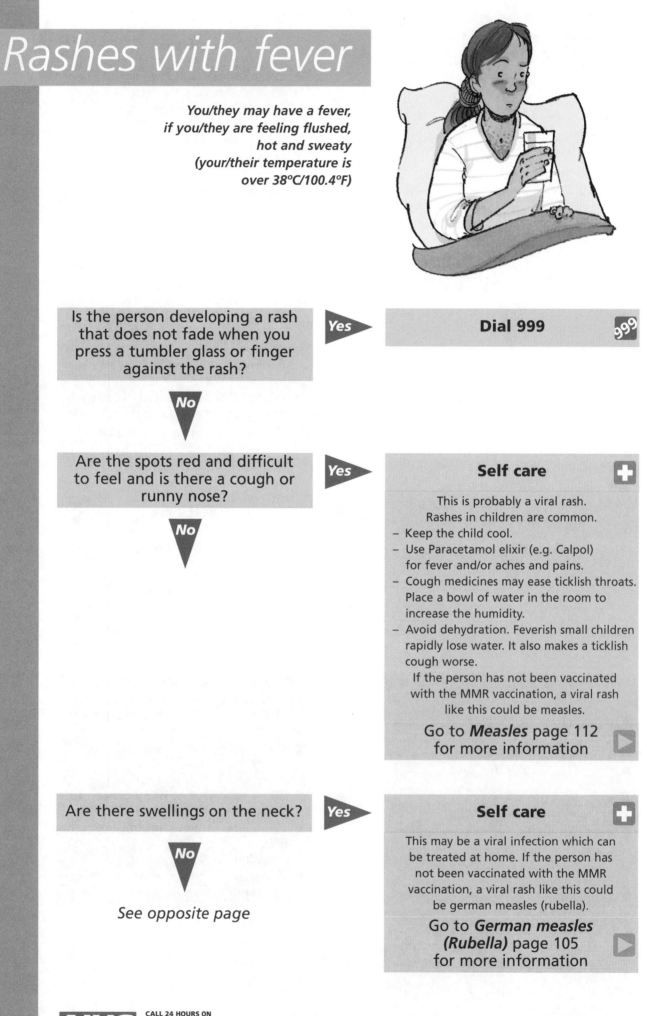

Is the person developing a rash that does not fade when you press a tumbler glass or finger against the rash?

Yes ▶ **Dial 999** 999

No ▼

Are the spots red and difficult to feel and is there a cough or runny nose?

Yes ▶

Self care ✚

This is probably a viral rash.
Rashes in children are common.
- Keep the child cool.
- Use Paracetamol elixir (e.g. Calpol) for fever and/or aches and pains.
- Cough medicines may ease ticklish throats. Place a bowl of water in the room to increase the humidity.
- Avoid dehydration. Feverish small children rapidly lose water. It also makes a ticklish cough worse.
If the person has not been vaccinated with the MMR vaccination, a viral rash like this could be measles.

Go to *Measles* page 112 for more information ▶

No ▼

Are there swellings on the neck?

Yes ▶

Self care ✚

This may be a viral infection which can be treated at home. If the person has not been vaccinated with the MMR vaccination, a viral rash like this could be german measles (rubella).

Go to *German measles (Rubella)* page 105 for more information ▶

No ▼

See opposite page

NHS CALL 24 HOURS ON
Direct 0845 4647

If you can feel the spot are they turning into small blisters?

Yes

No

Self care

It could be chicken pox. Intensely itchy, tiny clear blisters soon follow. Fresh red spots are usually seen next to blisters and crusts.

– Most children are free from chicken pox in less than two weeks.
– Dab calamine lotion on the infected spots which should ease the itching.
– Use cool baths without soap every three to four hours for the first couple of days. Add a few tablespoons of sodium bicarbonate to the bath water.
– Antihistamines are available from your pharmacist. These help reduce itching and promote sleep, so use them just before bed time.
– Paracetamol (e.g. Calpol) helps reduce the fever.
– Ice lollies help lower temperature and provide sugar and water while reducing the irritation of mouth infection. They can be used in children over 4 years old.
– If you are pregnant or think you could be, call **NHS Direct**.

Go to *Chicken pox* page 102 for more information ▶

Self care advice

■ A rash alone is unlikely to be serious.
■ Encourage the child to rest and observe closely for signs of illness.
■ Ensure the child is drinking plenty of fluids.
■ Paracetamol (e.g. Calpol) may be helpful if the child is restless.
■ Ask your pharmacist to recommend a cream that may provide some relief.
■ Calamine lotion will give relief for a short time.
■ 2 tablespoons of sodium bicarbonate (e.g. bicarbonate of soda) added to bath water may relieve any itching.
■ If the condition gets worse or if any other symptoms develop, call **NHS Direct**.
■ If you are still worried, call **NHS Direct**.

Before ringing NHS Direct or 999, it would be helpful if you think about the following and are ready to answer the questions if asked:
■ The symptoms (the questions you answered yes to)
■ Their temperature (if possible)
■ When they last had anything to drink or eat.
■ Any medicines they are taking at present
■ Any allergies you know of
■ Any serious illnesses they have had before.

We'll take the worry away

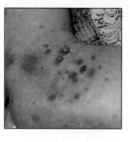

Chicken pox

Children exposed to the virus develop chicken pox 7 to 21 days later. In most cases there are no symptoms before the rash appears.

Symptoms

■ A mild fever, stomach ache and general malaise can occur a day or two before the flat, red rash appears. This generally begins on the scalp, face and back, but can spread to any body surface although it is rarely seen on the palms of the hands or soles of the feet.

■ Intensely itchy, tiny clear blisters soon follow.

■ Fresh red spots are usually seen next to blisters and crusts.

■ Most children are free from chicken pox in less than two weeks.

Causes This virus spreads quickly, especially between children. Sneezing, coughing, contaminated clothing and direct contact with the open blisters are all ways of catching this relatively harmless infection.

Prevention There is no vaccine licenced in this country at present.

Complications Complications are very rare, although chicken pox can occasionally lead to encephalitis (inflammation of the brain), meningitis or pneumonia.

Serious complications are more common in those children who are taking medicines such as steroids as they can lower the body's immune defence system. Speak to your doctor's surgery for advice now.

Self care

■ Use cool baths without soap every three to four hours for the first couple of days. Add a few tablespoons of sodium bicarbonate to the bath water.

■ Calamine lotion gives temporary relief.

■ Cotton socks on inquisitive hands will prevent too much scratching which can lead to infection.

■ Paracetamol (e.g. Calpol) helps reduce the fever. Do not give aspirin to children under 12 years of age.

■ Ice lollies help lower temperature, provide sugar and water and at the same time reduce the irritation of mouth infection. They may be used in children over 4 years old.

More information Chicken pox is no longer infectious after 5 days from the time the spots appear. The child may then return to school.

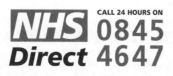

NHS Direct CALL 24 HOURS ON **0845 4647**

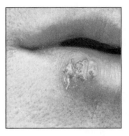

Cold sores (herpes)

Herpes is a virus which lives in nerve endings within the skin. It makes its presence felt around the corners of the mouth with crusty, oozing blisters.

Symptoms

■ A tingling, itchy feeling is usually felt just before the rash forms.

■ Tiny blisters appear, usually at the lips where they join skin.

■ The blisters become sore and itchy.

■ They then crust over and last about one week before disappearing.

■ They can return at any time.

Causes Kissing or other contact with someone infected with Herpes simplex. The virus is infectious, particularly when the blister is erupting.

Prevention There is not much you can do to prevent catching a cold sore other than avoiding kissing people who have obvious signs of it on their face. Once infected avoid sudden changes in temperature and sun exposure.

Complications There is a related form of herpes which can infect the genitals and which can be transmitted through oral sex.

Self care

■ Use simple painkillers such as paracetamol.

■ Use a lip salve with a high sun protection factor (SPF) before going into bright sunlight.

■ Aciclovir cream (e.g. Zovirax) will limit the outbreak if started as early as possible. Ask your pharmacist for advice.

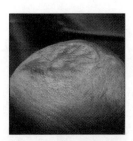

Cradle cap

A harmless white/yellow, waxy, scale which builds up on the scalp.

Symptoms

■ A thick white/yellow waxy scale builds up on the scalp. There is no bleeding or obvious irritation unless too vigorous attempts are made to remove it. There is no fever and the child is perfectly well.

Causes Like many other forms of eczema, the cause is unknown.

Prevention Routine cleaning will prevent it in most cases.

Complications There are no serious complications.

Self care

■ A form of eczema, it responds well to simply rubbing the affected parts of the scalp with olive oil. Leave it on over night before washing it off with a mild shampoo in the morning.

■ Shampoos are available from your pharmacist but you should try rubbing with olive oil first. Ask your pharmacist for advice.

We'll take the worry away

Cystitis

Women suffer most from this infection of the bladder which makes you pass water more often and may sting when you do. Men appear to get off lightly because of the greater distance between the anus from where most of the bacteria come and the urethra through which urine is passed.

Symptoms

■ Stinging sensation when passing water.

■ A feeling of needing to pass water very often.

Causes The most common cause is bacterial infection from the anus. Kidney stones. Diabetes.

Prevention Drinking plenty of fluids helps prevent cystitis in the first place.

Self care

■ Put a covered hot water bottle against your tummy to ease the pain.

■ Drink slightly acid drinks such as cranberry juice, lemon squash or pure orange juice.

■ Try a mixture of potassium citrate available from your pharmacist.

Note

– If you still feel infected after one day

– If there is any blood in your urine

– If you are pregnant

take a urine sample from your first visit to the toilet in the morning to the practice nurse. Use a clean, well-rinsed bottle.

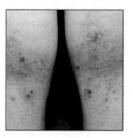

Eczema

Basically it is inflammation of the skin, for whatever reason or cause which produces dry flaky skin, more often on the inside of joints such as the elbow. It is more common in young people and old people. The term dermatitis is exactly the same thing but tends to be used when the eczema is caused by contact with a chemical or other substances.

Symptoms

■ Atopic eczema is an allergic condition. People who suffer from other allergies such as hay fever are also prone to eczema. It can affect any part of the body but the inside of the elbows, knees, wrists are the most common sites.

■ The dry flaky skin can come and go but tends to be worse in winter or cold weather.

■ Contact dermatitis can be very severe with the skin becoming deeply inflamed, leading to skin loss. The underlying deep skin looks red and angry. Infection is often the next step.

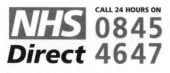

NHS Direct CALL 24 HOURS ON **0845 4647**

■ Seborrhoeic dermatitis is the name for eczema that affects the scalp and eyebrows. A thick yellow greasy scale builds up, leading to heavy dandruff.

Causes Atopic eczema is probably an inherited condition. The inflammation flares up as a response to some allergy although it may never be identified. Hair dye, nickel watch backs, jewellery and washing powders are all known to cause contact dermatitis in susceptible people. Seborrhoeic dermatitis may be fungal in origin, although it could equally be an extreme form of allergy affecting the hairy parts of the body.

Prevention It makes sense to identify and avoid those substances, materials or chemicals which trigger the eczema.

Keep the skin moist with emollient ointments. Your pharmacist will advise you.

Use a bath water additive which contains moisturising oils.

Complications Secondary infection may occur, particularly in very young children. Unfortunately, topical steroid creams, which can be so effective in treatment of eczema, also make the skin more prone to infection. Contact dermatitis can be so severe that the skin is lost in the affected area leading to infection and scarring. Not surprisingly this can be both intensely itchy and painful. Over use of steroids can be dangerous. Always follow the suggested dose on the package and ask your pharmacist for advice.

Self care

■ There is a wide range of products which will help stop the itchiness and keep the skin moist.

■ Topical steroid creams may be helpful. If the eczema is mild, ask your pharmacist's advice. If it's severe seek advice from your GP.

■ Scratching and itchiness can be reduced by keeping the skin moist and taking antihistamine tablets or medicine. This is useful for young children as it also has a mild sedative effect making for a better night's sleep for everyone.

Action – *Call NHS Direct but speak to your doctor if:*

– The eczema is spreading very quickly.

– The skin is becoming infected.

– There is severe pain.

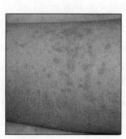

German Measles (Rubella)

Now uncommon thanks to the Measles, Mumps and Rubella (MMR) vaccine.

Symptoms

■ The person is rarely ill but will have a slightly raised temperature and swollen glands on the neck and base of the skull.

■ The pin head sized flat, red spots last around two days and need no treatment. Paracetamol will help reduce the slight fever.

We'll take the worry away

German Measles (Rubella) continued

Causes The virus is very contagious and will spread quickly in a population which is not immune.

Prevention Vaccination for girls and boys is both safe and effective.

Complications Very rarely the virus that causes German Measles (Rubella) will cause an inflammation of the brain (encephalitis). The real danger may come in later life if an unvaccinated woman becomes infected with German Measles (Rubella) while pregnant as it can affect the development of the baby. For this major reason alone both boys and girls should be immunised with this very safe vaccine.

Self care

■ Paracetamol will reduce the mild fever.

Hangovers

A hangover can be so bad you actually think there is something seriously wrong with you, especially if it is the first time it has ever happened.

Symptoms

■ Headache, nausea, tiredness and thirst are the commonest symptoms.

Causes Dehydration is the main cause. Alcohol acts as a diuretic stimulating the kidneys to lose water. Some alcoholic drinks contain toxins which act as mild poisons. Red wine in excess tends to cause headaches for this reason. Sleep while intoxicated is always poor as the alcohol interferes with the normal sleep pattern. This causes a feeling of not having slept the next morning.

Prevention Obviously the best way to avoid a hangover is not to drink to excess. Drinking a few glasses of water before retiring will also help. Switch to less or non-alcoholic drinks towards the end of the evening.

Complications Hangovers are rarely dangerous but routinely taking the hair of the dog to ease the symptoms can lead to alcohol abuse. People underestimate just how long alcohol stays in the blood stream after a night's drinking and may well be still over the legal limit for driving the next day.

Self care

■ Drink plenty of water, take paracetamol and if possible have a nap later on to make up for the poor quality of sleep.

Note If you are suffering hangovers regularly it is highly likely that you are abusing alcohol and may be becoming dependent on it. If people are commenting on your drinking, you are becoming defensive over it, your work or home relationships are suffering or you are drinking early in the day you should seek advice from **NHS Direct** or contact a support group such as Alcoholics Anonymous.

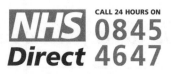

CALL 24 HOURS ON
NHS 0845
Direct 4647

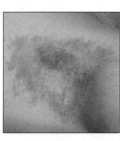

Heat rash

All babies and children will have a rash at some time (sometimes called 'heat rash').

Symptoms

■ It looks like a fine pattern of tiny red spots which come and go but tend to disappear if their temperature is lowered.

■ The baby will be perfectly well.

Causes A cold or a viral infection are the most common causes. Too many clothes or bedding will also cause it.

Complications If your baby gets too hot cool them down immediately by removing their clothes and keep them in a cool room.

Self care

■ No treatment is required other than lowering their temperature with paracetamol syrup (e.g. Calpol).

Hiatus hernia and Heartburn

This is the reflux, bringing up, of stomach acid into the gullet. The condition used to be more than just a nuisance before the appearance of modern drugs, which reduce the production of stomach acid.

Symptoms

■ Burning sensation (heart burn) behind the breast bone which is made worse by stooping or lying flat. There may also be an acid taste brought up from the stomach. There can be difficulty in swallowing with repeated reflux of stomach acid.

Causes The neck of the stomach rolls into the chest allowing stomach acid to pass into the gullet.

Prevention You can't prevent a hiatus hernia but you can ease the symptoms. You can prevent many of symptoms by:

– controlling your weight

– controlling how much you eat

– not smoking

Complications Constant acid irritation of the gullet can make swallowing difficult.

Self care

■ Avoid foods that trigger off attacks – such as rich and fatty foods. Take indigestion remedies (antacids) and drink milk to relieve the symptoms. Sleep with an extra pillow to stop the acid reflux.

We'll take the worry away

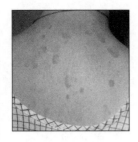

Hives / Urticaria / Nettle Rash

Symptoms

■ Hives are small often itchy, **raised** red spots which you can feel and are rarely serious unless combined with any breathing problems.

■ The rash will usually disappear in a few hours without any treatment.

Causes It is most often caused by certain foods and plants (e.g. nettles) but may be caused by a viral infection.

Complications Rarely the rash is severe and associated with breathing difficulties. This is an emergency. Dial 999.

Self care

■ A pharmacist may be able to recommend a cream or medicine that could provide some relief.

■ If there is any shortness of breath, dial 999.

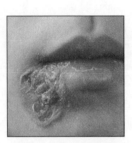

Impetigo

Bacterial infections of the skin are fairly common. Impetigo is more common in children but is also seen in adults. It is infectious but is no longer a serious threat, thanks to antibiotics.

Symptoms

■ It usually starts as a small red spot which gradually increases in size.

■ The top becomes crusty and weeps.

■ It is often found around the corners of the mouth and face, but can also be found on the rest of the body.

Causes It is infectious and is caught from direct contact with infected children or adults. It is also spread through sharing face cloths and towels.

Prevention Use separate washing materials.

Complications It spreads much more quickly in people who are generally run down with illness or stress.

Self care

■ Clean the spots with a damp tissue. Give painkillers such as paracetamol for any pain. Antibiotic creams are needed.

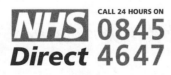

NHS Direct CALL 24 HOURS ON **0845 4647**

Indigestion

Indigestion is more common in middle aged people, after heavy meals or alcohol consumption and is often worse at night. Regurgitation or reflux is painful although rarely dangerous. Stomach acid escapes into the gullet causing chest pain. It can be mistaken for a heart attack. Severe reflux can occur with a hiatus hernia (see page 107).

Symptoms

■ Vague pain below the ribcage, extending into the throat.

■ Acid taste in the mouth.

■ Excessive wind.

Causes

– Classically after a heavy meal or drinking.

– 'Rich' food, often with a high fat content.

– Excessive smoking.

– A leaking valve at the neck of the stomach (hiatus hernia).

Prevention

– Avoid food which you know provokes an attack.

– Sleep with your upper body propped up with pillows.

– Avoid eating just before bed time.

– Eat small meals more often.

– Avoid aspirin and drugs like ibuprofen (non-steroidal anti-inflammatory drugs).

Complications
Most indigestion is harmless but annoying. The acid refluxing into the throat does not appear to cause any serious damage. The greatest danger is ignoring repeated attacks or confusing them with a heart attack. Obtain medical advice if your symptoms persist or get worse.

Self care

■ Your pharmacist will advise about indigestion remedies (antacids and other medicines).

■ Avoid taking large amounts of sodium bicarbonate (bicarbonate of soda) as this is turned into salt in the body.

■ A glass of milk before bed can help.

We'll take the worry away

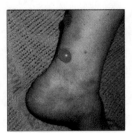

Insect bites and stings

At first, insect bites can be mistaken for more serious things.

Symptoms

■ If you look very closely you can generally see the small hole of the actual bite. The rash or individual 'spot' is invariably itchy and may swell, particularly if it is a bite from a horse fly (clegg).

Causes 'Midges', horse flies, bees, wasps, centipedes, ants, lice etc. The list is long but thankfully there are no killers within the UK.

Prevention Insect repellents work. If you suspect lice, ask your pharmacist for advice (see *Lice* page 112).

Complications Some people are strongly allergic to bites and stings and can be very ill. If there is any shortness of breath, dial 999. Bites can become infected by scratching.

Self care

■ Although itchy and sometimes painful they are rarely dangerous and need only some antihistamine or local anaesthetic cream from your pharmacist. Ask your pharmacist for advice.

■ The redness and swelling are usually due to the allergy rather than an infection. Antibiotics are rarely needed in the first 48 hours.

■ Call your doctor if the symptoms persist.

Irritable bowel syndrome (IBS)

Diagnosis is based on exclusion of any other conditions. There is no definitive test for IBS. It affects three times as many women as men. Symptoms can start at any age but predominate between 15 and 40 years. Stress and lifestyle are major factors. The cause remains unknown. It is rarely, if ever, fatal.

Symptoms

Along with excessive wind, the symptoms of IBS are:

■ intermittent constipation

■ diarrhoea

■ colicky tummy (abdominal) pain.

Causes The cause is unknown but it may be stress related.

Prevention

– Go for a high-fibre diet containing whole grain bread, rice and pasta.

– Eating plenty of fresh fruit can produce a remarkable long-term improvement in symptoms.

– Dairy products are often the bad guys. Try eliminating cheese, milk, chocolate, butter and cream from your diet for a few weeks to see if there is any improvement.

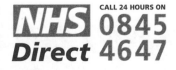

NHS Direct CALL 24 HOURS ON **0845 4647**

- Red meat, not just beef, can often seriously upset your bowel if you are prone to IBS.

- Use herbs known to alleviate the symptoms of IBS, e.g. peppermint.

- Stress can be a big factor.

- Exercise is valuable. It increases bowel activity thus reducing bloating and distension. Nicotine stimulates receptors in the bowel making IBS much worse.

- Small amounts of alcohol can actually help to stimulate gentle bowel function.

- Tea contains as much caffeine as coffee. Both, therefore, stimulate bowel action resulting in diarrhoea in the susceptible person. Coffee also contains an unknown substance that causes bowel cramps.

Self care

■ Drugs are the last resort and only have a temporary effect. Codeine relieves the spasm but can cause constipation. Peppermint oil is the basic ingredient of many drugs prescribed by your GP for IBS. Anti-diarrhoeal drugs and laxatives can help but long-term use of either is unwise.

■ The pain and discomfort of IBS can sometimes be relieved by a hot water bottle which fits nice and snuggly against your stomach.

However, see your doctor if:

- the home treatment doesn't work after two weeks

- you pass blood in your motions

- your bowel motions are very dark black or covered with mucus

- there is an unexplained weight loss.

More information For more information contact:

British Digestive Foundation
3 St. Andrews Place
London
NW1 4LB

We'll take the worry away

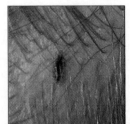
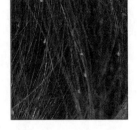

Lice

These tiny parasites can live on any hairy bits of the body. Female lice lay eggs every day. The eggs hatch in 8-10 days.

Symptoms

■ Nearly always they are completely harmless, but terribly itchy. Lice and their eggs (nits) can be seen on the hair shafts.

Causes Social status means nothing to lice. They are very common amongst children and infestation has nothing to do with dirty living.

Prevention

– Lice are easily caught from others. Avoid spreading lice by treating the whole family.
– Avoid lending or borrowing hats, brushes or combs.
– Keep hair clean.
– As lice can stay alive for two days when they are not on a human being, thoroughly clean clothes and hats which have been worn, as well as combs and brushes.
– To prevent lice comb the hair regularly while wet with a fine-toothed comb. Use a conditioner to make combing easier.

Self care

■ The safest and most effective treatment is daily combing with a nit comb. Use only conditioner and a nit comb or ask your pharmacist for advice.

More information Community Hygiene Concern, a government-funded organisation supply leaflets on 'Bug Busting'.
Help Line: 020 8341 7167

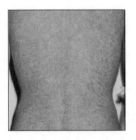

Measles

Children are most vulnerable to this highly contagious viral infection. With the MMR vaccination this is now very rare in the UK.

Symptoms

Symptoms usually develop in a well established order:

■ a mild to severe temperature of around 39°C/102.2°F

■ tiredness and general fatigue

■ poor appetite

■ running nose and sneezing

■ irritable dry cough

■ red eyes and sensitivity to light

■ tiny white spots in the mouth and throat

■ a blotchy red rash that starts behind the ears, spreads to the face and then to the rest of the body and lasts for up to seven days.

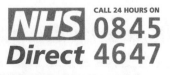

CALL 24 HOURS ON
NHS 0845
Direct 4647

Causes It takes around 10 to 12 days for the virus to make its presence felt after infection from another child. Physical contact, sneezing and clothing contaminated with nasal secretions all help to spread this infection.

Prevention Although immunisation rates are now very high you should isolate your child from other children if you think they may be infected. Immunised children and those who have already caught measles are virtually immune.

Complications Meningitis and pneumonia are rare but serious complications. More commonly, eyes and ears develop secondary infection which may need antibiotics from your doctor.

Self care

■ Once the rash starts it is a matter of treating the symptoms.

■ Check the child's temperature.

■ Use paracetamol elixir (e.g. Calpol) for fever and aches and pains.

■ Light sensitivity can be helped by reducing sunlight or electric lights in the room.

■ Use a ball of damp cotton wool to clean away any crustiness around the eyes.

■ Cough medicines are of little value but do ease ticklish throats. Try placing a bowl of water in the room.

■ Avoid dehydration. Feverish small children rapidly lose water. It also makes a cough worse.

■ Try one teaspoon of lemon juice and two teaspoons of honey in a glass of warm water.

■ Ideally, you should keep your child away from others for at least 7 days after the start of the rash.

■ After four days the child usually feels better.

More information To protect your child against Measles ensure that they are vaccinated with the MMR vaccination.

We'll take the worry away

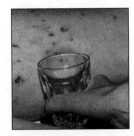

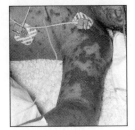

Later stage of the rash as it appears on a dark skin.

Meningitis / Septicaemia

A rare illness, it causes inflammation of the brain lining which can be fatal. Unfortunately the symptoms can be easily mistaken for flu or a bad cold. Worse still, it is more difficult to be certain with babies and young children. If you are not sure, you must call **NHS Direct***.*

Hib immunisation has reduced the number of people suffering from some types of meningitis/septicaemia. Unfortunately, we do not have vaccines for every type of meningitis/septicaemia, so we all still need to watch out for the symptoms of meningitis/septicaemia.

Symptoms

Babies under 2 years:

■ They can be difficult to wake.

■ Their cry may be high pitched and different from normal.

■ They may vomit repeatedly, not just after feeds.

■ They refuse feeds, either from the bottle, breast or by spoon.

■ Their skin may appear pale or blotchy, possibly with a red/purple rash which does not fade when you press a tumbler glass or a finger against the rash.

■ The soft spot on top of your baby's head (the fontanelle) may be tight or bulging.

■ The baby may seem irritable and dislikes being handled.

■ The body may be floppy or else stiff with jerky movements.

Remember a fever may not be present in the early stages.

Older children may have slightly different symptoms:

■ a constant generalised headache

■ a high temperature, although hands and feet may be cold

■ vomiting

■ drowsiness

■ confusion

■ sensitivity to bright lights, daylight or even the TV

■ neck stiffness – moving their chin to their chest will be very painful at the back of the neck

■ rash of red/purple spots or bruises which does not fade when you press a tumbler glass or finger against the rash. The rash may not be present in the early stages

■ joint or muscle pain

■ rapid breathing

■ stomach pain sometimes with diarrhoea.

Symptoms can appear in any order and not everyone gets all the symptoms.

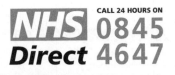

CALL 24 HOURS ON
0845 4647

Causes There are different types of meningitis which can be caused by either bacteria or viruses.

Prevention A vaccination programme has now started for Meningitis C for children and young people up to 17 years of age. It is safe and extremely effective. Some forms of meningitis do not, as yet, have a vaccination so the disease can still occur. It pays to keep an open mind.

More information The National Meningitis Trust provides free information to sufferers of meningitis and their relatives. Tel: 24-hour support line, 0345 538118. The Meningitis Research Foundation also operates a 24-hour helpline which provides help and information to the public and health professionals. Freephone 080 8800 3344.

Note People who have been in contact with someone who has had meningitis should contact a close relative of the patient to find out any instructions (from the hospital or the Director of Public Health) that they may have been given. Otherwise your doctor will be able to give you appropriate advice. Only those who have been in very close contact with the infected person are given antibiotics and vaccination.

Migraine

Migraine is common and runs in the family.

Symptoms

■ Visual patterns such as chequerboards or spots are often a warning of an impending attack. These can be quite debilitating, making the person sick and unable to concentrate.

Causes The exact cause is still not known, although there is some connection with the blood vessels of the skull. Certain foods appear to trigger migraine. Red wine, particularly Chianti, blue cheeses and chocolate are all culprits. Stress, the weather and even hormonal changes have been known to increase the suffering.

Prevention Avoid triggers such as red wine or blue cheese.

Complications The greatest danger from headaches is missing something more serious than the common causes. Irritability increases along with a shorter fuse. There is a greater risk of having an accident, as well as a risk of overdosing on paracetamol.

Self care

■ Light can hurt the eyes and lying in a darkened room helps for some people, although modern thought is to avoid such isolation and instead get on with 'normal' life. The attack can last from minutes to days. There are treatments available from your doctor which may reduce or even prevent a full blown migraine attack. Anti-inflammatory drugs (eg ibuprofen) can help ease the pain and are generally better than simple analgesics.

We'll take the worry away

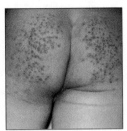

Nappy rash

Rashes in the nappy area are common but can be reduced in severity or avoided completely.

Symptoms

■ The rash is usually red, not raised and confined to the nappy area.

Causes It is caused by the irritating effect of urine and bowel motions. If they are cleaned away quickly enough, or the baby is allowed to have the nappy off for a while, the rash will not appear.

Prevention As far as is possible, change each nappy following soiling. Remember that urine can be every bit as irritating as faeces. Avoid disposable wipes containing alcohol or moisturising chemicals. Instead use plenty of warm water. As much as practical leave the nappy off, particularly any plastic pants. Dry, cool skin rarely forms a nappy rash. Reusable nappies should be washed as directed by the manufacturer. Avoid caustic household detergents.

Complications An angry red rash which does not respond or extends beyond the nappy area may be a fungal infection (Candida). You need an anti-fungal cream and an oral anti-fungal agent as it often starts in the mouth. Ask your pharmacist or doctor.

Self care

■ Promptly treat any rash appearing with ointment from your pharmacist.

■ Avoid talcum powder generally which can cake badly and cause even more irritation.

Peptic ulcers

Gastric ulcers affect the lining of the stomach and are more common in people over 40 years. Prolonged use of high doses of steroids, e.g. for asthma or rheumatic conditions, can cause a gastric ulcer. Even relatively small doses of anti-inflammatory drugs such as ibuprofen or aspirin can lead to an ulcer in the stomach in people who are susceptible. Duodenal ulcers which are found lower down in the abdomen are more common in men. They heal more easily than the gastric variety and usually develop just at the beginning of the duodenum.

Symptoms

■ The symptoms of peptic ulcers tend to overlap but a fairly general pattern is recognised.

Gastric ulcers

■ Constant pain or cramps can occur which are particularly bad after eating (eating tends to settle pain in a duodenal ulcer).

■ Indigestion remedies (antacids) often settle the pain but it invariably returns.

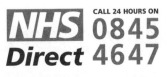

- Belching is common and embarrassing.
- Vomiting can occur.

Duodenal ulcers

- Most people know they have developed a duodenal ulcer at around 2 am when they wake with a pain like a red hot poker just above the belly button.
- Drinking milk can help but hot spicy foods make it much worse. Eating small amounts of food often relieves the pain.

Causes Ulcers may be caused by a bacterium called Helicobacter that lives in the stomach. Your doctor can check for this. Stress, smoking and alcohol abuse may also be causes.

Prevention Avoid smoking, excessive alcohol and 'rich' foods. Milk and indigestion remedies (antacids) do help.

Complications

Call your doctor if there is:

– blood or brown soil-like blood in your vomit

– black tar-like blood or fresh red blood in your bowel motions

– severe pain just below the rib cage

– dizziness when standing up

– a strong thirst.

Self care

- Most peptic ulcers will respond well to treatment with modern drugs which reduce the amount of stomach acid. You can also help ease the pain by using indigestion remedies or antacids.

Note If the pain has just started but is lasting more than a week, despite medicines from your pharmacist, call your doctor.

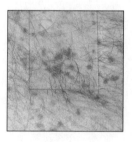

Purpura

Serious problems are rare. These irregularly shaped, dark red spots could follow an allergic reaction to infection or some disorder of the blood.

Symptoms

- The spots are not usually irritating, range from around pinhead size to a couple of centimetres (around one inch), tend to come and go and will not fade when pressed with a glass tumbler or a finger.

Causes Children between 2 and 10 years are most likely to be affected. There are a number of causes but anything that affects the ability of the blood to clot can cause this rash.

We'll take the worry away

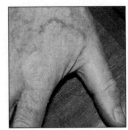

Ringworm (Tinea)

Ringworm (Tinea) can affect many parts of the body, particularly the groin and scalp.

Symptoms

■ It is most noticeable on bare skin when it is referred to as ringworm due to its characteristic appearance as a circular patch of red, itchy skin, which gradually increases in size.

■ There may also be red itchy areas around the base of hair shafts.

■ With scratching, these areas can bleed and become crusted with blood.

Causes It is not a worm, simply a fungus (Tinea).

Prevention Keep the area well ventilated and dry. Use a separate face cloth and towel – ringworm is infectious.

Complications Bacterial infection from scratching is common.

Self care

■ Keep the area well ventilated and dry.

■ Use a cream or special shampoo as recommended by your pharmacist.

Scabies

Although intensely itchy, scabies is rarely a serious condition.

Symptoms

■ Red lines which follow the burrows of the mite as it travels in the skin soon merge with the inevitable scratching. It is usually worse at night when the mite is most active.

Causes Scabies is caused by a mite which burrows just under the skin, often between the fingers, on wrists, elbows and the genital areas causing a red rash. It can only come from contact with infected people.

Prevention It is very difficult to prevent.

Complications Bacterial infection from excessive scratching can make the situation worse.

Self care

■ Ointments are available from your pharmacist. All of the body will need to be covered with the ointment for 24 hours and all clothing and bedding should be washed thoroughly.

NHS Direct
CALL 24 HOURS ON
0845 4647

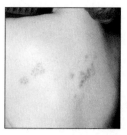

Shingles

One step up from cold sores, shingles is caused by a closely related virus. It is particularly nasty if the immune system is not working properly, during illness or while on treatment for cancer. It is rare to develop shingles more than once.

Symptoms

- A tingling itchy feeling precedes a painful rash.

- It is only found on one side of the body.

- It can develop over the next few hours or days into a painful set of blisters.

- It usually follows a narrow strip of skin, common sites include the chest wall, face and upper legs.

- A general flu-like illness often accompanies the rash which may persist after the rash has gone.

Causes If you have never had chicken pox you are very unlikely to develop shingles which is caused by the same virus.

Prevention Prevention is difficult, most people will develop the infection without realising where it came from.

Complications Although sometimes very painful, shingles is rarely serious. People who are suffering from any condition or medicine which lowers their resistance to infection can be quite ill. If it spreads onto the tip of the nose it may affect the eye and immediate attention from your doctor is recommended.

Self care

- Once the tingling sensation begins it is wise to start antiviral medicine, aciclovir (e.g. Zovirax).

- Simple painkillers such as aspirin and paracetamol help.

- Keep the rash area uncovered as much as possible.

- Try not to scratch the rash. Use calamine lotion to ease the itchiness.

- Pain which follows the disappearance of the rash can be reduced by cooling the area with a bag of ice.

See your doctor, especially if:

– the outbreak of blisters occurs near your eye or at the tip of your nose

– you also have a sore red eye

– the sores have not healed after 10 days

– there is also a high temperature

– you suffer from some other serious illness.

More information Although it is possible to treat the infection with aciclovir (e.g. Zovirax) it is important to start treatment as soon as possible when the itchiness first starts. Once the rash is well developed, aciclovir is of no great value.

We'll take the worry away

Smoking & lung cancer

Lung cancer was rare until tobacco hit the scene. Some things will not go away in a puff of smoke:

– This is the most common type of cancer in men with over 100 new cases per 100,000 men diagnosed each year in the UK. 31% of all deaths from any cancer are from lung cancer. 30,000 men develop it each year compared to 14,000 women, but women are catching up. More women than men smoke, most of them young women.

– The peak age for lung cancer is between 65 and 75 years; it is relatively rare below the age of 40.

– Only 8% of people survive lung cancer.

– Tobacco smoking in its various forms is the single biggest cause.

– The more cigarettes smoked and the younger the age at which smoking started, the greater the risk.

– Cigar and pipe smokers have a lower chance of developing lung cancer, but their risk is still higher than for non-smokers.

– Inhalation of tobacco smoke by non-smokers – known as passive smoking – has also been shown to be a risk factor for lung cancer.

Symptoms

You should go to your GP if you:

■ have a persistent cough

■ have coughed up blood

■ have an increasing shortness of breath.

Causes Smoking causes lung cancer. Full stop.

Prevention Giving up smoking, or better still, not starting in the first place makes sense. Around 100 people die every day from lung cancer. Half of all heavy smokers will never reach 70 years of age. Even light smokers only have a 60% chance of survival until the age of 70. There are now four times as many non-smokers as smokers so you can do it if you really put your mind to it.

Self care

■ Nicotine patches can be purchased over-the-counter from a pharmacist at the cost equivalent to one packet of cigarettes per day. These can be very successful in easing the craving for nicotine.

■ Get in touch with self-help groups or organisations which supply information.

■ If you can't do it for yourself, do it for your partner or kids.

Quit plan:

■ Set a day and date to stop. Tell all your friends and relatives – they will support you.

■ Like deep sea diving, always take a buddy. Get someone to give up with you. You will reinforce each other's willpower.

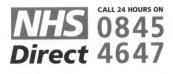

NHS Direct CALL 24 HOURS ON 0845 4647

■ Clear the house and your pockets of any packets of cigarettes or tobacco, papers or matches.

■ One day at a time is better than leaving it open ended.

■ Map out your progress on a chart or calendar. Keep the money saved in a separate container.

■ Chew on a carrot. It help you do something with your mouth and hands.

■ Ask your friends not to smoke around you. People accept this far more readily than they used to do.

More information

QUIT
102, Gloucester Place
London
W1H 3DA

Smokers Quit-line: 0171 487 3000 (9.30 am-5.30 pm daily)

Note

– Within 8 hours all of the poisonous carbon monoxide produced by smoking has been washed out of your blood. At the same time the oxygen levels return to normal.
– Within 24 hours your chances of a heart attack, much higher while smoking, begin to decrease.
– Within 48 hours the nerve endings destroyed by smoking begin to re-grow. Smoking stops you coughing by killing off the nerves which control the cough reflex. You may well find yourself clearing your lungs better after two smoke-free days. Your sense of smell will become stronger as will your taste. Many people put on weight after stopping smoking for just these reasons, they enjoy their food more.
– Within 3 days spasm of lung tissue decreases making breathing easier. Lung capacity increases.
– Within 3 months your circulation has improved, walking becomes easier and even your liver begins to improve. Most of the de-toxification of the nasties absorbed from smoke takes place in the liver.
– Within 5 years your risk of lung cancer has dropped dramatically. Some doctors say by up to 50% and the risk will return to normal within 10 years.

We'll take the worry away

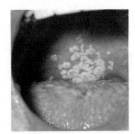

Thrush in the mouth.

Vaginal thrush

Candida albicans is a fungus which should not normally be present in large numbers in the vagina. For various reasons it can grow rapidly and cause thrush.

Symptoms

■ A creamy thick white vaginal discharge.

■ Itchiness and irritation.

■ Pain or burning after passing water.

Causes

– A prolonged course of antibiotics.

– The oral contraceptive pill. Hormonal changes preceding the period.

– Steroid treatment.

– Diabetes.

– Immune system problems.

– Sexual intercourse with an infected man.

Prevention After being on the toilet, wipe from front to back. Change underwear frequently, particularly after exercise. Choose cotton rather than nylon pants. Avoid harsh soaps, they kill the good bacteria which prevent thrush.

Complications Thankfully there are few serious complications of thrush. It can, however, make life very miserable. Sex is painful, as is passing water.

Self care

■ Eat live yoghurt and apply it to the vaginal area. It will replace the missing Lactobacillus which prevents thrush.

■ Ask your pharmacist for anti-fungal preparations.

■ Your partner may need treatment as well.

See your doctor if:

– thrush does not disappear after self care or keeps coming back for no apparent reason

– if the discharge changes in smell or appearance

– there is any abdominal pain.

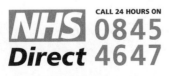

CALL 24 HOURS ON
NHS 0845
Direct 4647

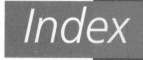
Index

We'll take the worry away

Index

We'll take the worry away

NHS Direct CALL 24 HOURS ON **0845 4647**

Index

We'll take the worry away

127

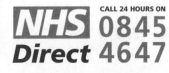
CALL 24 HOURS ON
NHS Direct 0845 4647